Dr Clive Wood is a freelance science writer who was originally trained as a biochemist and physiologist. For the last ten years he has been concerned with the relationship between behaviour and disease, and has been involved in the organization of several conferences on the topic. After being trained in California in the assessment of Type A behaviour, he has more recently been involved in a research project at Oxford University into the relationship between Type A and the cardiovascular system. He has given lectures and seminars on heart disease at the Universities of Oxford and Cambridge, and is a member of Linacre College, Oxford.

Clive Wood

Living in Overdrive

Fontana Paperbacks

First published by Fontana Paperbacks 1984

Set in 10 on 12 point Linotron Plantin
Made and printed in Great Britain by
William Collins Sons & Co. Ltd, Glasgow

To Nancy
with the laughing face
and the video recorder

Contents

Acknowledgements   9
Preface   11

1 Slipping into Overdrive   17
2 Enter Type A   29
3 What Stops the Pump?   57
4 Effort, Distress and Your Adrenals   68
5 Superpong and Hot Responders   97
6 Raising the Odds   115
7 Cholesterol Revisited   136
8 Aerobics and Beta-blockade   151
9 Relaxing is a Skill   182
10 From Relaxation to Meditation   204
11 Out of Overdrive   224
12 Saving Your Own Life   256

Selected References and Notes   271
Index   277

Acknowledgements

For permission to reprint copyright material, I am grateful to the following authors and publishers:

D. A. Bernstein and T. D. Borkovec, *Progressive Relaxation Training: A Manual for the Helping Professions*, Research Press, Champaign, Illinois, 1973.

Daniel J. Levinson, C. N. Darrow, E. B. Klein, M. H. Levinson, B. McKee, *The Seasons of a Man's Life*, Alfred Knopf Inc. and The Sterling Lord Literary Agency, © 1978, Daniel J. Levinson.

Dr Herbert Benson, 'The Relaxation Response', excerpted by permission of the *New England Journal of Medicine* (296; p. 1153; 1977).

Preface

It's just ten years since a book appeared that changed the direction of my life. *Type A Behavior and Your Heart* was written by two San Francisco cardiologists. It described a pattern of self-destructive behaviour to which many of us are prone, a set of mindless, stereotyped reactions that we go through many times a day. If it really gets hold of you, the pattern has two consequences. First, it produces a frustration and anguish that makes you feel as though you're going to explode. And, second, it brings you closer to a heart attack.

When I read the book in my late thirties I was no stranger to the first of these. I'd often felt the desire for a sort of 'temporary death', a total switch-off to let the tension flow back to wherever it came from. But I wasn't looking for the real thing. A heart attack, particularly a self-induced attack, really did seem the ultimate stupidity. The book suggested ways of avoiding it. I followed them. I still do.

This book is an attempt to go a little beyond the scope of that original study and to look at the problem of what I've called *overdriving behaviour* from a slightly broader perspective. It's broader because the idea of overdrive goes further than that of Type A. The two overlap but they may not be the same. It's broader too in the way it tries to relate this type of behaviour to the many other risks that also increase our chances of coronary disease.

The most important single fact to have come out of all the research done on heart disease since World War II is that it doesn't have any single cause. A whole set of factors – raised cholesterol, high blood pressure, cigarettes and so on – all make their contribution. So too does the way we act – our own particular pattern of behaviour. We don't yet understand how these risk factors interact with each other, and the fact that the mix is different in different cultures, and perhaps even in different individuals, certainly doesn't help.

But while all physicians agree that coronary disease is 'multi-factorial', that doesn't stop many of them from concentrating almost exclusively on the factor of their choice. Of course, it's natural enough to emphasize those features you happen to be most interested in. When I teach classes of students, I'm sure I do the same myself. Unfortunately, the different interest groups are in danger of becoming isolated as there's a real tendency for the cholesterol or blood pressure or behavioural specialists to concentrate so exclusively on their favourite risk factor that they downgrade all the others.

Let me give you an example: on the same shelf of my bookcase are two chapters on heart disease, written by leading experts, sincere men both of whom I know and respect. The first, on diet, says quite clearly that 'in the longer term only an overall dietary improvement is likely to reduce the amount of coronary and other arterial disease, since diet is the fundamental factor'.

The other is equally plain: '. . . no matter what your diet, no matter how vigorously you exercise and how valiantly you shun cigarettes, if you have not altered your Type A behavior then the probable chief cause of your first heart attack is still operating to produce another one.'

If anything, these partisan positions have hardened in the last couple of years with the publication of results from large and elaborate trials which were designed to reduce risk factors and hence reduce coronary mortality in selected groups of people. Despite the effort and the costs involved, they have had only limited success. Their opponents say, 'We told you so; you're looking in the wrong place.' Their supporters say, 'Oh no, the facts are clear enough; the trials simply didn't manage to prove them.' They then carry on as though nothing had happened.

So we're left in a remarkable situation. With only three exceptions, we have no foolproof evidence that reducing our risk factors is going to reduce our coronary death rate. We just act as though we had. The exceptions are cigarette smoking, *very* high cholesterol levels and Type A behaviour in men who've already had one heart attack. This is true despite the much-publicized fall in heart deaths that has occurred in the USA during the last fifteen years. One American in five is now surviving the disease that would previously have killed him, but no one fully understands why.

In this book I have tried to look broadly and without (many) irrational biases at this multi-factorial disease. If I have spent more time on the physical risks than you might expect in a book on self-destructive behaviour I hope the reason is clear. To give them less attention is to create a picture so distorted that it helps no one.

Even so, my main interest is in our behaviour and in the physical damage that it can do to our bodies. So I've gone to the same lengths to explain how each of us alters his or her biochemistry by getting hassled or by hassling other people. It's the sort of biological mechanism that fascinates physiologists like me. But if that's all it was – a set of reactions that we could look at but couldn't do anything to influence – then it would hardly be worth a book. Fortunately for all of us, we can change our biochemical responses by learning to change the way that we behave, and just like other risk factors, it's only common sense to do so. I hope to convince you too that the change is worth making but whether you agree or not will depend, among other things, on how desperate you've become.

So this is a book about how we react and respond to our surroundings. What I haven't written is yet another book about stress. It's true that the notion of stress has been immensely useful over the last thirty years in helping to explain how diseases arise that have no obvious physical cause. But the concept has got badly mauled. Even the word itself is used by different specialists to mean at least three different things. Stress can either be some threat or danger out there in our environment, or the way that we assess such a threat, or the way our bodies react to it. It depends on the expert you talk to. There is now even a distinction made between *eustress* which is essentially pleasant and *distress* which isn't.

Because of all this confusion I decided some years ago not to use the word at all. And I must say that I haven't missed it. When you do find it mentioned elsewhere in this book, it will be when I'm quoting from other people. As to the difference between eustress and distress, I share the view that eustress is a challenge you can readily cope with. Distress is one that you can't. Overdrivers are frequently distressed. They seek out situations that have a potential to create distress, though what they are actually looking for is a feeling of mastery.

So the element of distress crops up many times because overdrive is not only bad for your heart. It's really no fun either, once it gets hold of you. For both of these reasons, physicians and psychologists are finally trying to do something about it. And this book is an attempt to chart their progress so far.

When I was half-way through it I mentioned it to a friend of mine, a university teacher in his mid-thirties who is no stranger to the down-side of overdrive himself. 'As far as I can see,' he told me, 'books like that end up pushing either booze, yoga or God. Which one gets your vote?'

The answer certainly isn't booze, though moderate drinking is supposed to benefit your cholesterol; nor is it God, though there is evidence that regular churchgoers have fewer heart attacks than atheists; it includes yoga, or rather, the relaxation that goes with it, and a lot of talking to yourself.

The two words that sum it up best are *insight* and *redirection*, the two basic needs, I suppose, that keep analysts in business. But psychoanalysis may not have much to offer the overdriver. Counselling has, but that's a different story. So has group therapy (if you can talk about therapy for a group of people who aren't ill). But mostly it's something you can (and have to) do for yourself.

At about this point in a preface it's usual to say that a book like this could not have been written by one person on his own. And of course it's true. That's not because of a lack of data. You can get the facts from the scientific journals (though they may be a year old by the time they appear). What you can't do sitting in any library is to get a *feel* for the facts, for what's important and what's not. Nor can you find out what's happening *today*. But worse than that, you can't pick up on the sheer excitement of it all without doing what anyone who calls himself a scientist loves to do – going off to talk to other scientists about what they're doing and what they're thinking.

And so my gratitude goes out to dozens of research workers in Europe and the United States for the help and stimulation that they have given me in putting parts of this story together. They really are too numerous to mention, without you getting awfully bored, but of those whose work is referred to in the book, I am particularly grateful to Ad Appels, Herbert Benson, Malcolm Carruthers, Margaret Chesney, Nancy Fleischmann, Meyer Friedman, David Glass, David Jenkins, David Krantz, Bob Levy, Chandra Patel, Lynda Powell, Ray Rosenman, Ethel Roskies, Carl

Thoresen, Redford Williams and Steve Zyzanski.

My thanks are also due to my many friends in Oxford who let me bounce ideas off them. The ideas usually came back in better shape. I want to express particular thanks to Jane Irving, Derek Johnston and Alvin Ross for their constant stimulation. But neither they nor anyone else I have named are responsible for the conclusions I have reached, nor even for the routes I took to get there. The misunderstandings and misconceptions are all my own, but then again, so was the pleasure of doing it.

Oxford
March, 1984
Clive Wood

1. Slipping into Overdrive

Here are six questions about your approach to life. Try to answer them as honestly as you can. You may find the results revealing.

- Are you hard driving and competitive?
- Are you usually pressed for time?
- Are you bossy or dominating?
- Do you have a strong need to excel in most things?
- Do you eat too quickly?
- Do you get upset when you have to wait for anything?

If you have answered 'yes' to most of these questions then I can make a few predictions about you, based on a recent eight-year study of nearly two thousand people who live the way that you do.

You probably find that life is full of challenges and you often need to keep two or more projects moving at the same time. The chances are that you have been to college, that you have a management job and that you bring work home at night. You think that you put more effort into your job than many of the people you work with, and you certainly take your work more seriously than most of them. You get irritated easily, and if someone is being long-winded, you help them get to the point. You also have trouble finding the time to get your hair cut.

And there's one other thing. You are about twice as likely to have a heart attack as someone who takes a more easygoing approach to life.

The mention of heart attacks probably makes you think that surveys like this only apply to men. After all, men up to middle age in Britain and America have about four times more coronaries than women do. But women suffer too, if they adopt this same hard-driving, competitive, time-urgent lifestyle. Working women living this way are twice as likely to develop coronary disease as those who are more relaxed.

You might expect things to be different for housewives, since living at home should cause less hassle than going out to work, and as a group, housewives in this study were more easygoing. But some felt the same time pressures as women with outside jobs; the sense that things would get out of control unless they tried all the time to keep on top. Those who felt this suffered three times as much heart disease as those who didn't whether, they looked after an office or a home. And women with children, who were married to blue-collar workers and were holding down clerical jobs at the same time, had the highest heart disease risk of all.

The beginnings of your hard-driving behaviour go right back to childhood. In school you got recognition and perhaps prizes for being quick and bright, for being an achiever, for competing with others and *for winning*. You probably went on from school to get a series of increasingly better jobs against pretty stiff competition. They were jobs where you had to care about the results, where you constantly had to push things forward and get things done. In your present job you also feel some conflict, either with time or with other people. Some of those you work with don't seem able to grasp the simplest ideas, and they often put a brake on what you're trying to achieve. The conflict may not erupt every day. You pride yourself on being able to keep the lid on. But it's always there, under the surface.

Deep down, you have an urge to take control, not because you are a better organizer than anyone else (though you may be) but simply because if you're in charge then things are going to work. You simply won't let them do otherwise.

Do you recognize yourself yet, the man or woman who leads from the front? If so, you also have to know about the price-tag for staying there. Because you feel you have to be on the look-out for things going wrong all the time, you live your whole life in a state of readiness. You're always prepared to move some situation along, or to stop it slipping backwards. It's a way of life that increases your risk of ending up prematurely exhausted and burnt-out, and doubles your chance of inviting a coronary, the stage beyond burn-out, and a terminal stage for one victim in every two.

But you may say, 'That's not me. I've never wanted to control anything except my personal life. Just the opposite. I get jumpy and overstretched when things start to move too fast. I just want to insulate myself from all that.' Fine, if you can, but very few of us are able to isolate ourselves from a way of life that keeps us more aroused than we ever wanted to be, at least not if we've got a living to earn. You may never have wanted to call the shots. But having to live and work with those who do can make the cost just as high. If you let it.

I'm going to suggest that you don't have to let it. Many psychologists and cardiologists now believe that the way that we see our world and respond to it has profound effects on our bodily and mental health. In this book I shall try to summarize some of their research, especially their belief that by changing our behaviour we might be able to avoid both burn-out and heart attacks. Their findings are starting to suggest ways that the hard-driver – the overdriver – might use to stop himself from cracking up.

The question is does he want to? I don't rate anyone's success in changing your behaviour very highly if you are under thirty-five, hooked on an overdriving lifestyle and haven't had a coronary yet. You probably believe that keeping on the move, keeping the adrenaline flowing, and letting the bastards have it now and again is the key to whatever success you may have achieved. Then there's the recession to consider. A good job these days is hard to find. If you've got one, and you've worked hard to make it what it is, you're not likely to put it on the line because someone says it may do you harm in five or ten years. Your monthly cheque does you good right now, and no one believes that unemployment improves your health.

If you do feel that way then all I have to say is, 'Go for it – and good luck.' You have to establish yourself in a competitive world, and success gives you excitement as well as money. It's not time yet for you to start worrying about what it's doing to you. But that time will come – probably in your late thirties when you're well enough advanced to afford the luxury of looking back at how you got there. In the meantime I suggest you read on. You'll need to know about overdrive, if not this year then maybe next.

The results will surprise you, because what the research is showing is that, apart from damaging your heart, overdrive is not the keystone of success that you think it is. Quite the reverse. Much of it actually holds you back and stops you from achieving what you really want to do. For that reason alone it's worth making changes. I'm not suggesting that we should stop rewarding effort, simply that we may be able to achieve the same result at a lower cost. There are good reasons for believing that working hard and moving fast aren't dangerous in themselves. The breakthrough is in coming to see the rest of our overdriving behaviour for what it is.

Most dangerous of all is the way that many of us live in a constant state of over-arousal. Our nervous systems are continually over-reacting – a way of life that for convenience, I have called *overdrive*.

But perhaps you're not a victim. Some people do say to

me, 'You're quite wrong about all this stress and tension. Personally I thrive on pressure, I love it; without it I'd be dead.' The last one to tell me so was a retired professor of cardiology, an expert in his field. He had run a hospital department with a world-wide reputation. Not only did he have a staff of first-class physicians to do much of the work. He also had almost total freedom to run his department the way he wanted. Life for him was a stimulating challenge, a constant source of interest and reward. He worked longer hours than many men half his age but rarely was he in the slightest danger of losing control of any situation. If that's pressure, who wouldn't thrive on it?

But anyone who has worked on a production-line knows pressure of a different kind. He knows the relentless pace that is set, not by any action on his part, but simply by the speed of the machine. The job may be mindlessly boring but you simply can't 'switch off'. You are forced to be constantly on the look-out for anything going wrong. So it comes as no surprise that production workers pay a price, at least as high as any white-collar overdrivers. When the demands of the job are high, but your freedom to make decisions is low, heart disease is one result, and in industrial societies like the United States and Western Europe, it is the blue-collar workers who have most of the coronaries. Of course, if you do spend your day behind a machine, you are still likely to become just as angry as any executive when you have to queue in a post office or deal with a check-out clerk. And your hostility affects your arteries in just the same way.

There's an irony in all of this. It may be possible to separate the effort that goes into a job from the distress that it causes. At the Karolinska Institute in Stockholm, a research team has been working for many years on the human cost of production-line labour. They came to suspect that the key feature in deciding whether a particular job is distressing or not is the amount of control that the worker has over what he is doing. To test their ideas they had volunteers in a laboratory do a series of jobs that needed vigilance and repetition, quite similar to work on the production-line. The researchers found that negative job features like boredom, impatience and irritation didn't go along with job involvement (as measured by effort or concentration) as long as the volunteers were allowed to work at their own pace. Being able to predict and control the speed of their work and being confident that they could keep up with it, changed a series of monotonous and distressing tasks into a job that made the workers feel pleasantly challenged.

The same Swedish group were among the first to point out that designing the job for the worker might actually make him more productive. But the message will be slow in coming across. Retooling our major industries has a low priority at a time when many wonder how manufacturing is even going to survive the next two decades. Job satisfaction is something of a luxury when the first priority is to keep the job, satisfactory or not. In fact we're going to have more reason for adopting an overdriving lifestyle in the mid-1980s than ever we did even in the 1960s or 1970s. Overdrivers thrive on competition and there's going to be no shortage of that before the year 2000.

To stop the overdriving pattern from ruining our lives we need to learn two simple lessons. The first is that achieving your aims doesn't mean having to live in a constant state of over-arousal. You don't have to be hostile, competitive and impulsive to the point of neurosis. Nuclear specialists talk about developing a 'flexible response capability'. It means responding to each level of threat with just as much reaction as necessary – no more, no less. In the same way, the overdriver has to learn to meet different types of challenge with a graded set of responses. It simply makes no sense to live your whole life at condition red.

The second lesson is even simpler. Each of us has to be

responsible for our own welfare. In other words, you have to save your own life. By the time things are bad enough to get the doctors involved, you're well on the way to disaster. And that's what this book is about – helping yourself.

Do you think I am exaggerating the overdriver's problem? George and Irving don't.

George was forty-seven and living in Washington when his first heart attack hit him. For two or three years he had had odd chest pains and he quite often got short of breath. He thought if he ignored the pain it might go away, but it didn't. It got worse. When someone suggested he should see a doctor he laughed: 'What, me have a heart attack; are you kidding?' The months before the attack had been stormy. He had broken up with his lover and moved out of the apartment. His mother had finally died from cancer of the throat. Her end was slow and painful – and almost as painful to watch. There were money problems too. His real-estate business had never run smoothly, but recently he seemed to have to be there twelve hours a day to keep it moving at all.

George didn't remember much about his coronary. He did remember waking up in intensive care and asking the doctors a dozen times what was happening. Eventually one of them told him his heartbeat was uneven, and he seemed to have suffered a heart attack. Only later did he find out that the same doctor was telling his sister Lois that he had suffered a massive coronary. If he lived through the here-and-now (which was uncertain) his prospects of long-term survival were pretty poor.

But he did live through it. The day he left the hospital was the happiest of his life. So it was for his fourteen-year-old daughter. All Donna wanted was to have her daddy home. The reality turned out to be different for both of them. George had always seen himself as a Princeton half-back, virile, fast moving and 'capable of taking anything they can dish out'. Now he was trapped in an apartment with his daughter and widowed sister. Donna went through agonies trying to help, but he threw all her efforts back in her face. He was a cripple, and he hated her for knowing it. Nothing she could say got through to him and soon she was terrified to say anything at all.

The doctor told her that her father's reaction was normal for someone with his condition, but she didn't care about what was normal. All she wanted was to have a father she could love. She dreaded being asked home by her friends, for if she had to ask them back they would discover her horrible, embarrassing secret. Unable to hate him, she started to hate herself and for the first time in her life she knew what it was to feel guilty. Her school work started to suffer. Wherever she went, whatever she did, the burden of her father went with her.

Lois got the same treatment but she had her own life to lead. She tried to act as though nothing had happened. She would come home in the evening, tidy round and make supper, whistling a tuneless noise just loud enough to blot him out. She spent whole mealtimes steering the conversation away from anything that could cause the slightest offence. Robbed of any excuse to blow up, George would create one and blow up anyway. Without saying a word, Lois would clear the table, wash the dishes and go to her room.

After 'years of inactivity' (actually twelve weeks) George was allowed to return to his office part time. Almost at once he had a blazing row with his partner, an easygoing family man who had been running things. ('What do you mean it's a slack time? You've got to go out and *make* the business for Christ's sake.') The partner left. Within a month things started to fall apart. For George, the failure had nothing to do with bad management. It was just another sign of his lost virility and his insecurity became unbearable. Just before he died he described himself as 'panic-stricken and hopeless.

One of the living dead. Fifty years old, going on seventy-five.'

He was actually fifty-one when the second attack struck him. The doctors said he must have died within seconds of feeling the pain. Donna and Lois mourned him for as long as they could, but they were both surprised how difficult it was to sustain their grief beyond the day of the cremation. Now they have a binding, unspoken agreement. They never talk about him at all.

Irving had his coronary when he was a little older than George. He was fifty-two when he first started to notice the heartburn that came on walking the three blocks from the parking lot to the café he owned in mid-town New York. It was worse in cold weather. To be on the safe side, he took his wife's advice to see the doctor who was already treating him for high blood pressure. The electrocardiogram (ECG) showed nothing unusual and both men agreed that it must have been something he had eaten. Irving had seen the same doctor for years and had complete confidence in him. 'You've always been like a father to me,' he used to say. Father or not, the pains got worse. Irving went back, this time for an exercise ECG, taken while he was stepping up and down on a box. Again nothing. Three weeks later he was having breakfast when the heartburn came on 'a hundred times worse than anything I'd ever known before'. The pain in his chest spread to his left shoulder and ran down his arm. He was starting to sweat. His wife phoned the doctor, Irving's father figure. He was at his club. She phoned the hospital. They asked her to describe the symptoms, and when she did so they said, 'You'd better bring him in.' When Ruth recalls the occasion, she still feels nauseous.

All his life Irving had owed nothing to anyone. So who needed an ambulance? The Toyota would get them there faster. It had to be heartburn. There had been a few heart attacks in the family. Two of his uncles had gone that way, but it couldn't be happening to him. He didn't smoke, he wasn't fat, and he certainly got plenty of exercise running about the café fourteen hours a day (Sundays too – he was proud of that; none of the competition had the stamina to open on Sundays).

Somehow the car found the hospital, but the car park was full. The closest lot was half a mile away – the longest half-mile he'd ever walked. He staggered through the door and collapsed in the lobby. He remembers waking up in intensive care. The machines he was hooked up to both reassured and frightened him. He was getting the benefit of all the latest gadgets but it was like living in a space capsule. However, his most vivid memory of intensive care has nothing to do with the electronics. Instead he remembers, for the first time in his life, a feeling of warmth and reassurance from knowing that his wife or son would be with him most of the time.

Once the immediate crisis had passed, Irving was moved into coronary care. There were no space-age monitors but the two-patient rooms were staffed by extra nurses. 'They watch your every move,' he told his son. 'They even uncross your legs for you. Trouble is, it's like being on death row.' Every few days a patient in the unit would die and like the inmates of a prison, everyone else seemed to know immediately. Irving went through more depression than he could ever remember in that room. He found himself crying almost every day, something he had not done since he was a child: 'I've always been too damn busy,' he used to say with some pride. But here with the closeness of death, everything changed. Everyone on the unit shared the same thought – maybe I'm next. One night Irving's room-mate collapsed in his bed. A flurry of nurses rushed the screens around him and Irving heard himself screaming, 'Frank, don't do it, don't die on me.'

But Irving himself didn't die. He made what the doctors called an excellent recovery. Of course he had to convalesce, and there were many things he would never be able to do, like going back to heavy work or even carrying a bag. Now his wife brought the shopping from the supermarket. He went with her, but he walked behind so that people wouldn't wonder why he was letting her take the packages to the car. She didn't mind. She understood his problem, and far from being a burden, she was pleased to have him home during the day. Not that she had too much time at home herself, for it was her job that now became vital.

Irving never wanted his wife to be the breadwinner full time. But he knew he could never return to the café. It was like losing a child when he sold it for half what it was worth. Finding another job wasn't easy either, but with some of the money he managed to enrol to study accountancy. College was tiring, but they arranged his course so that he only went three days a week, with time to rest in between.

Irving's attitude to work has changed completely. Today he says: 'I am not going to hurt myself by rushing around. I'd rather take care of myself than jeopardize my health. It's far more important to me than money.' He still lives in fear of a second, perhaps fatal, attack and he always will. He did have a recurrence of his chest pain, but it passed off in half an hour. This time he let his son drive him to the hospital. The doctors told him that not enough blood was reaching his heart. Such episodes would come and go, but they were not as serious as the heart attack that nearly killed him.

When someone asked him whether the rest of his life had changed since that day at breakfast, his reply was immediate. 'Absolutely,' he said, 'one hundred per cent. Physically, psychologically and socially. I've been able to adapt to it because of my wonderful family, my good friends and the people I've been able to get along with. But I wonder about anyone without friends and family like mine. What would happen to them? An illness such as mine couldn't be handled alone.'

George and Irving were two in a million, just two of the million men to suffer a heart attack in the United States every year, and at over a hundred thousand, attack rates are similar in England – higher if anything. George was one in half a million. They are the American men who die from it, more than half of them before they reach hospital. Both of them show the typical signs of the coronary-prone personality. The commonest and most dangerous is denial. George and Irving were both sure it could never happen to them, and most of us feel that way. We've all read the statistics and we don't think they lie. We just don't think they're relevant. Take the most frightening one of all: *a third of all deaths among American men between thirty-four and sixty-four are caused by cardiovascular disease*. Not so frightening perhaps if it means that two-thirds are due to something else. You have to go eventually, and two chances out of three aren't bad odds for a betting man.

Then look around. How many of these fatal statistics did you know personally? One, perhaps, two, three? Four or five if you are unlucky, it depends on your age. 'It's not that I don't believe the figures,' George or Irving might have said. 'It's just that they measure someone else's problem.' But they'd both have been wrong. And the odds suddenly change when you're the one holding the short straw.

2. Enter Type A

There is a story told among American physicians which rivals the tale of Benjamin Franklin and his kite. It too has several versions, but one of them goes like this.

One day in the early 1950s an upholsterer came to re-cover the waiting room seats at a doctor's office in San Francisco. When he had finished he asked what sort of practice they had there. They said they were both cardiologists. 'I was just wondering,' he replied, 'because only the front edges of your seats are worn out.'

The physicians were Dr Meyer Friedman and his then partner Dr Ray H. Rosenman. The office was in the Mount Zion Medical Center where Friedman at the time was director of the Harold Brunn Institute. The story is told in their prize-winning book *Type A Behavior and Your Heart*. The book was published twenty years after the event, but Friedman recounts the incident vividly. It was one of several happenings that changed his thinking about the whole problem of heart disease.

At just that moment the two cardiologists were studying the many reports that had been published on cholesterol and coronary disease, so as to condense all the findings into a review. In 1955 when the review was published, most physicians (and their patients) believed that dietary fat and cholesterol were probably *the* major cause of coronaries. So dietary advice was the cornerstone of treatment. Even today, Friedman advises his cardiac patients to keep their fat intake to an absolute minimum. 'Take the fruit pie,' he says, 'not the cheese.'

But as Rosenman and Friedman reviewed what had been written about cholesterol in the diet, they noticed some facts that didn't fit. For example, if white women had the same fat intake as their husbands (and a small diet survey among volunteers in San Francisco showed that they did) then why were they less coronary prone? Friedman couldn't believe the then popular idea that they were protected by their sex hormones, because black women weren't. There had to be other factors working.

It was the wife of a San Francisco executive who gave him the answer. 'If you really want to know what is giving our husbands heart attacks,' she said, 'I'll tell you. It's stress. The stress they get in their work. That's what's doing it.' As for her own husband: 'I have to give him a martini when he comes home at night, just to get his teeth unclenched.'

Friedman was polite, but sceptical. The idea that work pressure could bring on a heart attack seemed far-fetched in the diet-oriented 1950s. But it was not unthinkable. Here and there scattered about the medical journals of the past half-century, there had been suggestions that the way the heart patient confronts his world might have an effect on his health. They decided to test the suggestion. At least, they decided to find out whether two groups of people at the sharp end, business executives and their doctors, agreed with it.

They sent out a questionnaire to 100 executives in three Californian corporations, and to a similar number of physicians who treated coronary patients. The letter asked quite simply what they thought had caused the heart attack that had recently been suffered by a friend or patient of theirs. They gave ten or more causes to choose from, including cigarette smoking, lack of exercise, worry or anxiety, and a suggestion of their own described as 'excessive competitive drive and meeting deadlines'. The executives were in no doubt. More than seven out of ten said that deadlines had been at least partly responsible for their friends' attacks. Amazingly enough, most of the physicians thought so too, though hardly any of them were advising their patients about it.

If these beliefs about competition causing heart attacks were true, then highly competitive, time-pressed individuals, constantly up against deadlines, should have more heart disease than those who were relaxed and easygoing. So Friedman and Rosenman asked a group of people in high-pressure corporations – newspaper offices, advertising agencies, TV stations – to nominate the most intensely driving and competitive person they knew. These nominees were then invited to come for a clinical examination, and the majority agreed. Finding a comparison group of employed men in San Francisco who were free from this drive for achievement and recognition was more difficult than they had expected, but eventually they managed to recruit enough, mostly municipal clerks and members of an embalmers' union.

The two groups were asked whether they currently suffered from pains in the chest, whether they had ever had a heart attack as far as they knew, and if they had felt chest pains in the past which might have been due to minor attacks that had gone unnoticed. Blood samples were taken for cholesterol measurements. They were also given an electrocardiogram to see if their heart rhythm was normal, or whether it showed any cardiac disease. The results were striking. The men from the high-pressure environments, whom the cardiologists described as 'chronically harassed by their various commitments, ambitions and drives', had higher cholesterol levels in their blood serum than the other volunteers. They also had seven times more coronary heart disease, judged by their medical history or ECG findings.

The researchers were careful to stress that not all groups of hard-driving men are going to show a sevenfold increase in disease. These particular individuals had been chosen because they showed this type of overdrive in its most extreme form. At the same time, nineteen of the twenty-three who were found to have coronary problems were completely unaware of them.

The effects of time pressure weren't confined to men. Rosenman's comparison of two groups of women also showed those with the time-urgent behaviour pattern to have higher cholesterol levels and four times as much coronary disease as those who didn't.

This link between hard-driving behaviour and raised cholesterol came as something of a surprise. To look at it more closely, the two cardiologists decided to examine a group of tax accountants over a period of six months, both before and after 15 April, the final day for completing the tax returns that they had agreed to prepare. They also examined some corporate accountants who had an additional work deadline for filing corporation accounts in January. All of them agreed to give blood twice a month and to keep a diary of what they ate and how they felt. Accountants made perfect subjects and most of their diaries were kept meticulously.

Their serum cholesterol levels in the first two weeks of January were much higher than in February or March, and those accountants with January deadlines showed cholesterol rises then too. Each accountant was asked when he personally felt that he had been under the greatest pressure. In nine cases out of ten, the time when he felt himself most harassed was the time of his greatest cholesterol rise. One could almost use cholesterol as a barometer of distress.

In 1958, when these findings were first made public, few physicians were ready for them and they were largely ignored. There was a cool reaction among delegates at a convention of the American Heart Association when they reported their results.

In fairness to the AHA, when the Californian results first

saw the light there was still a vital question to be answered. It was interesting enough to look at the frequency of heart disease in particular occupations, executives for example. But was it possible to *predict* in a group of normal healthy men, which of them were actually going to develop coronary disease in the future? All the best-designed heart disease studies then going on were trying to do just that. In Framingham, Massachusetts, for example, volunteers were examined at a screening visit and then followed up over the years. The value of that first examination in predicting future disease or death was then judged by recording what actually happened to them as time went by.

For their ideas to gain recognition, Friedman and Rosenman had to tackle the same crucial questions. Did their pattern of time-urgent, competitive behaviour have any value in *predicting* those who would suffer from coronary disease? And if it did was it really news, or did it simply mean that the future victims were high on other risk factors like cigarettes or cholesterol as well?

In 1960 they embarked on their most important investigation, one that was to take them more than ten years to complete. The Western Collaborative Group Study as it came to be known (WCGS for short) was a major undertaking. First they succeeded, by a combination of publicity and persuasion, in recruiting over three thousand men, all initially healthy and between the ages of thirty-nine and fifty-nine. They worked for various corporations around San Francisco Bay like Standard Oil, Lockheed and the Bank of America. Most of them had clerical or executive jobs and would have considered themselves to be middle or upper-middle class. The majority were earning salaries (even in 1960) of $10–15,000 and some were earning up to $25,000. About half of them were found to be hard-driving, aggressive and ambitious, the predictors that the study was designed to test. And of course some of them had other heart disease risks as well – raised cholesterol, high blood pressure, heavy smoking – all of which were measured at the same time.

After the initial examination, the WCGS volunteers were followed up for an average of eight and a half years. During that time more than two hundred of them suffered some form of coronary heart disease.

And what were the predictors? As expected, raised blood pressure and serum cholesterol, heavy smoking and coronary disease in the family all increased the chances of heart disease developing during the course of the study. The hard-driving behaviour pattern also predicted future disease. Indeed, it predicted all forms of coronary disease – chest pain, heart attack (better known to physicians as *myocardial infarction*) and sudden coronary death. A hard-driving man living in a chronic state of conflict was found to be about twice as prone to most of these disease states as someone more relaxed and easygoing. For recurrent infarction (a second heart attack) the risk was increased more than five times.

But how do we know that these two hundred-odd cases of coronary disease in the WCGS weren't due to something quite different? After all, hard-drivers tend to smoke more cigarettes, to have higher blood pressures and to push their cholesterols up more than other people. The answer is simple. There are now powerful statistical programmes especially designed to disentangle the effects of all these different influences. Running for minutes or sometimes hours on the computer, these programmes show up the effect of the factors we are interested in – in this case competition and hostility – while allowing for anything else that might interact at the same time. And even when all these other influences are allowed for, the hard-driver, the *overdriver* (and it was Meyer Friedman who first used the term) still carries a doubled risk simply from being the way he is. The other factors add to his problem. To be more precise, they multiply it.

Are we talking about you? Let's take a closer look. When Rosenman and Friedman really got down to examining their coronary patients, they found a group of men who seemed to be engaged in a relentless contest to obtain an unlimited number of things out of life. But the things they were chasing – money, prestige, position – were not really defined. The patients were rushing after something they could not describe in any clear way. And rushing was the operative word. Everything had to be done as quickly as possible. Quicker still, if they could find a better way of doing it.

Not only did their driving force compel them to work long hours and take work home in the evenings and at weekends. It also meant that they were invariably involved in doing two or three things at once. Winding up one project, beginning another, planning a third; reading reports, writing memos and making phone calls. The same was true at home. Coronary-prone patients would frequently read in the bathroom: a common enough habit perhaps, but some of them would try to shave at the same time. And many believed that driving to work was the only time to dictate their letters. This compulsion to use every minute of the day in 'purposeful activity', to pack as many goal-directed actions as possible into the available time, was obvious enough to the two physicians. But the patients themselves had lived with it for so long that many of them didn't even notice it. To them it was the way that any normal person behaved.

Their other striking feature was hostility. Someone who drives himself through life trying to get more done than he did yesterday – to get to the office earlier, to draft a more binding contract, to have a more creative staff meeting – is bound to be frustrated by anyone who blocks his lane on the highway, interrupts him with some trivial phone call, or arrives half an hour late for an appointment. Small wonder that he turns his anger on them. Hell for him really is other people, with their massive incompetence that stops him getting through all the things he has to do today.

Some of his aggression is turned inwards too. How stupid he was not to see that the agency was going to lose the account, or that the bank loan was going to be called in. How he kicks himself that he didn't catch the earlier plane; that he didn't pack a second copy of the agreement; that he had to waste two days in bed with a pulled hamstring.

Hurry and aggression are the cornerstones of his life. Friedman once suggested that the perfect heraldic emblem for the coronary-prone patient (I suppose a company logo comes closer today) was a clenched fist holding a stop-watch. I might suggest a motto to go with it. What about: 'Get out of the way, I'll do it myself'?

Now you might say that a lot of us are like this some of the time. Most of us have periods when we are forced to rush faster than we want to, and when we find ourselves being rude to people when we never intended to. It happens when we have to get something important done – moving house, settling into a new job, getting a full tax rebate. But the patients whom Friedman and Rosenman first described did it all the time. For them, it was a way of life.

What the two cardiologists saw, patients who sat on the edge of their chairs ready to rush into the doctor's office then rush out again, was something that few psychologists ever seemed to have noticed, and certainly none had labelled. And what label could they put on this behaviour? It wasn't really neurosis, although it had many neurotic features. It wasn't any other well-known psychological cluster like compulsion or obsession either, though it had elements of both. And so they decided not to put any fancy label on it at all. Instead, they suggested that the whole pattern should simply be described as *Type A*, and that's what it has been known as ever since. And the behaviour of those who didn't carve a quick and hostile furrow through life? They called that *Type B*.

Type Bs share many of the same characteristics as Type As, they are not simply As in reverse. They too have to earn a living and sometimes they have to compete. They're not passive, ineffective dummies. They simply don't react as often as Type As, or in the same exaggerated way. The Type B is a person with special strengths, but he also has particular problems of his own.

So how do you recognize a Type A? For many of us that means how do you recognize yourself, and the question is not as naive as it sounds. Many of those locked into the pattern have spent so much time in purpose-directed 'doing' that their image of themselves and their own make-up is completely distorted.

Recognizing the fully blown Type A (the so-called A1) is all too easy. You may know one, be married to one or you may be one. He walks quickly and is alert and aware. He looks you in the eye with an expression that can be anything from direct to downright hostile. When he sits to talk to you he is often perched forward on his seat with his body held tense. His speech is frequently explosive, with the key words driven home in such a way that you are left in no doubt about their importance, and his long sentences get faster towards the end.

If you interrupt him, then interesting things happen. He may let you finish, then go back to where he was ('As I was saying . . .'). More likely, if he is in full flow, he either says 'If I may just finish this point . . .' or else he simply talks right over you. How often in business or education do we hear two A1s supposedly in conversation, but actually conducting two solos. Seeing them galloping through a discussion, with clipped, staccato questions receiving instant abbreviated replies, is like watching a game of tennis played very close to the net. The problem is even worse on the telephone, where there aren't any visual clues for guidance. One Type A's impatience to get it all said means that he can easily miss

most of what the Type A at the other end of the line is trying
to tell him.

For anyone who suffers from the pattern, any delays are
simply intolerable. He will often start replying to your
question long before you have finished asking it. If he thinks
you are slow in getting to the point, he will help you with a
suggested word or phrase, and if that doesn't do it he will try
'Yes, mm, right' or 'I see' to get your sentence finished.
Talking to a fully fledged Type A can be an unnerving
experience. All the time you feel that he is shifting you up
to his pace, and resisting can be difficult. If you are at all
Type A yourself you will find that you are racing with him.
You may come out of the interview feeling strung up and
wrung out at the same time.

The fully developed Type B isn't difficult to recognize
either. He moves more slowly and holds himself looser than
the Type A. He is more inclined to smile, and when he does
so it is not with the Type A's tight-lipped grimace. When he
looks your way you don't feel that he may be sizing you up
for a fight. He will sit back in his chair and his body will relax
as he listens to what you have to say. Some seconds may pass
before he starts to reply. You don't feel that you have to keep
up with his pace. You don't feel that the two of you are
competing, and the reason is that unlike Type A, the Type
B simply doesn't care what you think of him.

It may not be difficult to tell an A1 from a B today. The
work has already been done. But in the early days in
California, there were many mistakes and false starts in
trying to get some measure of just how strong the pattern was
in any particular individual. Friedman had long been
interested in the psychology of leadership, particularly
among the military, and so one early attempt involved
reading a speech that might have been given by a general to
his troops before a battle. You could easily imagine John
Wayne or George C. Scott, the chin-strap of his one-star

helmet hanging loose, telling his battle-hardened brigade: 'You and me and every goddamned one of us are going to lick hell out of whoever stands in our way . . . First we're going to smack them hard with mortar fire, understand? . . . Let the bastards feel it get hot . . . make ashes out of them . . . After the mortars I'll tell you when to advance, and when I give the signal you don't crawl, you *run* forward. Remember it's your skin or theirs. Hey, one more thing. Good luck.'

The subjects read this speech to themselves until they were familiar with it, then recited it out loud under 'battlefield conditions'. At the same time their output was recorded and turned into an electronic voice-print. Type Bs delivered it smoothly and quietly, but Type As, even reading it to themselves, were in their element. Fully committed to getting out there and winning, their voices carried that explosive punctuation which is so much their hallmark, and the speech trace showed it clearly.

Another method in the early days was to measure the patient's breathing by putting an expandable belt around his chest. When bored or distressed, many Type As clench their fists and this too was measured by having them hold a hollow rubber ball. If they squeezed it, the pressure of their grip was registered. After being wired up, they were subjected to a tape recording of a woman relating a lengthy and completely pointless incident. In such conditions, time-conscious Type As can be expected to wriggle and squirm. And they did.

But both methods had drawbacks. The voice-prints needed elaborate equipment, too complicated for screening hundreds of subjects. The strain-gauges feeding the 'polygraph' recorder (like a Type A lie detector) were also too cumbersome for routine use. And though the polygraph worked well with private patients who followed the doctor's instructions to listen to the tape, when it was tested with Type A volunteers it didn't work at all.

The reason took some finding, but it was really quite simple. Rather than remaining bored and annoyed by the frustrating story on the tape, most Type As simply 'switched off'. They stopped listening and got on with thinking their own more important thoughts. It's a common pattern. Most of us have come across the Type A manager who seems to be giving you his attention but is thinking about other things and who may actually be signing letters at the same time. It is alleged that a famous Secretary to the Cabinet Office often used to say to his subordinates, 'You don't mind if I get on with reading these papers while we're talking, do you?'

The polygraph experience taught the researchers how difficult it is to predict just how distressed anyone is likely to become. Distress depends on whether you have some way of coping with the situation – in this case simply switching off and getting on with something else inside. If so, you may be able to protect yourself against disturbances that others would find intolerable. But without an effective means of coping, some people will crack up under what you or I would regard as very little provocation. Give an A1 newspaper editor twenty minutes to redesign the front page, and although he won't like it he'll get on and do it. Make the same editor spend twenty minutes writing the alphabet and his distress will start to show. He's simply not equipped to cope with under-employment.

Rosenman and Friedman used this fact in developing their best measure of Type A. They came to realize that the behaviour usually appears in particular circumstances. It becomes most noticeable when the individual is faced with a challenge or when he sees some threat looming up which might interfere with what he is trying to achieve. It doesn't matter whether the threat is real or not, what matters is that it is real *for him*. Such a threat usually comes from someone else – a supervisor, colleague, waiter, cab-driver or bank clerk – anyone with whom he has to interact. So if this interaction could be arranged – if the subject could be challenged in particular ways, perhaps within the context of an interview – then anything he saw as threatening might activate his underlying Type A behaviour. This was the line of thinking that eventually led to the most sensitive of Type A tests – the so-called *structured interview*, or SI. I say 'so-called' because it is not really an interview at all, although it looks like one. It is largely an exercise in provocation.

The SI is conducted by an interviewer specially trained to bring out the Type A pattern. Originally she (and the best interviewers proved to be women) recorded the subject's responses at the same time, but this was difficult to do. So interviews were recorded, first on audio and then on video tape. Replies could then be analysed and scored at leisure. During the setting up of the WCGS, for example, well over a thousand such interviews were recorded, which subsequently formed a 'bank' both for further research and for training other interviewers and scorers. The method has seen changes over the years and different variations exist, but the most widely used form of the interview only takes about fifteen minutes to complete. Volunteers are frequently surprised that it is so short. 'Is that all?' I am often asked after I have taken them through it. The content of the interview has also changed, but today it includes some twenty to thirty questions.

For example, a subject is asked whether he is satisfied with his present job level; whether he would describe himself as a hard-driving, ambitious kind of person, and whether he plays games for the fun of it or because he is really in there to win. His answers give a measure of his competitive drive. Hostility is revealed by such questions as 'When you get angry or upset, do the people around you know about it?' and 'What irritates you most about your work?' And the speed at which he lives his life is judged from questions like 'Do you always feel anxious to get going and finish whatever you have to do?'

Next comes impatience. New interviewers are sometimes amazed by the response they get to a simple question like 'When you are in your automobile and there is a car in your lane going far too slowly for you, what do you do about it?' I have heard agonized replies delivered through clenched teeth about how you can avoid being held up at all if you plan your journey to the last detail and are prepared to switch lanes at each intersection. One executive used to curse his driver for not understanding the Type A's golden rule, that you have to keep the wheels turning no matter what happens. The same man would boast that as a result of these carefully thought-out strategies he often arrived at his destination ten minutes early. 'What do you do then?' 'Oh, I just sit in the car and wait.'

But if conditions on the highway can bring out frenzied impatience, so too can a question like: 'How do you feel about waiting in line?' Type As simply hate queues. Many of them put real effort into planning exactly the right time of day to go to the bank, the post office or the supermarket, that magic moment when the queue is at its shortest.

All of these questions are clearly provoking. They dredge up memories and make the subject relive situations in which he may feel distinctly uncomfortable. The content of each answer is given a score, say from 1 to 5, to measure how Type A he really is in each of these circumstances, and the total score is added up.

But the interview is also provoking in another way. It contains a number of pointless questions, asked slowly and hesitantly, about what time the subject gets up, how often he has his brakes checked, even whether he develops his own films. The Type B subject will let the interviewer stumble to the end of the question. Only then will he reply, perhaps after thinking for a few moments about his answer. Not so the Type A. His answer is there – 'Six o'clock . . . Twice a year . . . Never' – before the question is half asked. The style of his replies gives an added measure (some would say the most important measure) of his Type A behaviour: the loudness and explosive delivery of his responses, the speed and acceleration of his replies and the shortness of the gap between question and answer, all contribute to the total score.

Some subjects are so hostile that they turn it on the interviewer. 'What do you mean by that?' or 'Why are you asking me all this?' Others actually compete to control the interview itself. They pitch in either with long rambling replies, or short abrasive jibes.

So the SI looks at both the content of their answers and the style of answering. But Friedman and his associates also concentrate on a third dimension. They believe that what the subject actually *does* during the interview is also important for assessing whether he is Type A or not. Other experts are not so convinced. After all, the WCGS only used audio tapes, with no visual input. But while the question is being resolved, these mannerisms still are very revealing.

For example, some Type As jiggle their knees up and down, or tap their fingers on the side of the chair. Their whole posture is tense and they may emphasize their replies (often forcefully) with sudden explosive gestures. Often the Type A subject will nod vigorously while he is speaking, as though to drive his point into your head, and some have a characteristic way of drawing back the corners of their lips, a nervous tic which, when you first see it, reminds you of Humphrey Bogart. All of these body movements are assessed from the video, and the SI generally reflects the subject's responsiveness to provocation.

Measuring Type A on a numerical scale – a sort of Type A ruler – is fairly recent. In the 1960s when the WCGS was being set up, the assessment of subjects from the interview was much cruder. They were either Type A or B, with each type subdivided once more to give four sub-types from A1 to B4. Some 10 per cent really did seem to be in the middle, showing the characteristics of both As and Bs. They were known as Type X.

These categories are still used and are still valuable, but they are not ideal. Human beings can't easily be fitted into ready-made boxes. Most of our characteristics – height, weight, blood pressure, cholesterol levels – lie on a smooth curve, high at one end and low at the other. They simply don't belong in three or four pre-ordained slots. Some investigators realized this, even early in the 1960s, and started to look for some simple way of expressing Type A with a number, just as you can express body temperature with a figure like 98.4°. At the same time, they were looking for a method that didn't need an experienced interviewer – there weren't many of them around. A questionnaire that the subject could complete for himself might be the answer. And if it could be scored by computer, then so much the better.

Hence was born the Jenkins Activity Survey, or JAS, originally a 64- (now 78-) item questionnaire that you can fill in for yourself and return by mail for scoring. Named after one of its authors, Professor C. David Jenkins, who was then at Boston University Medical Center, the JAS orginally tried to duplicate the findings recorded at the interview in a simplified form. Since much of the interesting information in the interview comes not from what the subject actually says, but from the way he says it, and, it seems, from what he is doing while he is saying it, no one would expect the JAS to replicate the interview completely. And indeed it doesn't. It gives an assessment based on what you believe to be the truth about yourself, and because Type As are often blind to their own driving self-destruction, their answers, even when honest, may be wrong.

Even so, the JAS has been of great value. It seems particularly to measure the urge for speed, competition and achievement. It can be given to hundreds of people at a time. When compared with interviews carried out on some of the original WCGS subjects, it was found to have an independent power of its own in predicting new cases of coronary disease. Not only that, but it has proved to be a particularly strong predictor of recurrent infarction, and the JAS score may even predict the amount of blockage in a patient's coronary arteries.

It has another value as well. By analysing the replies in a particular way, the overall concept of Type A can be broken down into three separate components, each approached by a different set of questions.

The first is called *Speed and Impatience*, a measure of time-urgency assessed by questions like 'Do you ever have trouble finding time to get your hair cut or styled?' The second, *Job Involvement*, measures the subject's dedication to his work by enquiring, for example, whether he would accept promotion to a higher job level without any increase in pay. The third, *Hard-Driving and Competitive*, explains itself. A question to reveal it is: 'Would people you know well agree that you take your work too seriously?' Put all these scales together and you have the overall JAS Type A score. How high it is depends on your sex (Type A is less common in women); your age (higher values are found in younger men); your level of education and occupation (the higher they are the higher you score); and also, it seems, your nationality.

So how high are you? To get an accurate answer you would need to be tested properly, but a few levels for different occupations may give you a clue. Remarkably high JAS scores were achieved by a group of eighty-three NASA executives in Washington. Hardly surprising perhaps, when you think about the approach and sheer attack required to design, build and launch a multi-million-dollar rocket, complete with lunar module and astronauts. And you have to do it by a particular date, with the news cameras of the world looking over your shoulder – an ideal combination for generating Type A.

But the NASA scores are not the highest. They are beaten by a group of Californian physicians on an American Heart Association postgraduate course – the very men who are supposed to be giving patients advice on how to deal with their Type A problems. And higher again were fifty-seven attorneys in what were described as 'high-ranking' law firms in Virginia. This surprises no one who has ever dealt with such men. Certainly it will come as no surprise to the lawyers themselves. I remember an interview when one corporate attorney paid another what he no doubt regarded as the supreme compliment. 'In court,' he said, 'he's pure combat.'

There are some groups of American men in high-status jobs who have scores below the average of the WCGS population, but not many. For example, air traffic controllers in New York and New England scored distinctly in the B direction, but senior officers and flight personnel in the Air Force didn't. Lower scores in the USA are generally found in lower occupational levels. A study of food store workers in Georgia found truck drivers, market assistants and labourers to be very Type B, more so than assistant managers or clerks. Managers and foremen, in contrast, were distinctly Type A and the administrators in charge of them all were amazingly so, with scores even higher than the attorneys.

Type A scores outside the United States seem to be lower than in America itself. British civil servants, Belgian postal and telegraph workers, even a cross-section of employed men in Finland where heart disease is rife, all scored far below the Western Collaborative average. It may be that European men simply don't feel themselves to be under as much pressure as their American counterparts, although it is also possible that they feel it without showing it in such obvious ways.

I have no doubt that Type A will prove to be an

international syndrome, but I would not be at all surprised to learn that middle-aged American men are well ahead of their competitors in the league tables. It is surely no accident that the pattern was discovered around San Francisco Bay, at a time when it was one of the most competitive industrial complexes in the world.

There have been other attempts to measure Type A, either more quickly or more cheaply than the SI or the JAS. The best known is the questionnaire with which I started Chapter 1 (remember: 'Are you hard driving and competitive?'). These questions come from Framingham, a town that became the Peyton Place of heart disease research for over two decades. By the mid-1960s it had become clear to the National Institutes of Health, which supported the Framingham Study, that as well as looking at physical risks, a number of psychological factors might also be examined at the regular bi-annual examinations of Framingham volunteers. So short questionnaires were drawn up, not only for Type A, but for other factors like tension, anger and ambition. These questions were asked of over one thousand, eight hundred subjects between 1965 and 1967. They were then followed up over the next eight years to see how their scores on these scales (like their blood pressure and cholesterol levels) also predicted any future coronary disease.

No one imagined that the ten-item Framingham Type A Questionnaire (from which I selected the six more important questions) would capture the whole pattern revealed by the structured interview. Even so, the Framingham scale, the ultimate in cheapness and simplicity, seems to have surprising predictive power, at least in assessing the distress that goes with Type A. Among white-collar (but not blue-collar) men under sixty-five, Type A behaviour measured by the scale was associated with a threefold increase in the risk of coronary disease.

Women in the same age group who developed heart

disease also had significantly higher Type A scores. As we saw, working women under sixty-five were almost twice as likely to develop coronary disease if they were Type A, and among Type A housewives the risk was increased threefold. Working in the home seems to give you no protection if you suffer from the Type A pattern, but neither does there seem to be much foundation for the idea that coronary risks necessarily increase when women take up outside employment.

There is going to be a lot more discussion about the findings from Framingham, not only about whether the wife's level of education or job status might influence her husband's risk (it seems that they do), but more especially whether Type A behaviour increases coronary risks only for men in white-collar jobs. It may take five years or more to decide whether Type A is largely an American disease and a middle-class complaint. But in a way it hardly matters. There are quite enough middle-class Americans with coronary problems to make its treatment a number one priority, and I suspect that many British men will need the same.

The question that both physicians and psychologists have been asking ever since the Type A pattern saw the light, is whether it needs a detonator. Is it something people carry around wherever they go, or does it only exist when they are hassled? Maybe the Type A only gets that way at work, and perhaps at weekends or on holiday he loosens up.

The thinking behind the structured interview was that Type A is brought out of people by some challenge or threat, and we now have a fairly clear idea of the kind of threats that do it. Imagine a group of volunteers in a psychology laboratory being given a mild electric shock or having their hands plunged into a bucket of iced water. In response to such treatments, or even while waiting for them, most volunteers will show an appreciable increase in pulse rate or blood pressure. But their responses will not tell you who is Type A or Type B. Both generally react to much the same extent.

But if you challenge their *self-esteem*, by giving them something to do and telling them it is important for them to do it both quickly and well, then the Type A often shows himself. His heart rate and blood pressure are likely to increase more than the Type B next to him, even though both of them are performing the same task (say a piece of mental arithmetic) with the same set of instructions. It seems to matter more to the Type A to get it right. He doesn't necessarily perform any better, but he certainly puts more into it.

Psychologists also love to have their subjects play TV games (the subjects like it too), to see how they will react to conflict. In one variation, two opponents in different rooms can communicate by sending messages to each other's TV screens. To play the game, they have to agree either to cooperate or to compete with each other, but if they see any advantage in doing so they can also cheat. By competing, a player can gain points, but without his opponent's cooperation he also runs the risk of losing them.

When two Type Bs play this sort of game they frequently cooperate and both gain the same number of points. So it is when a Type A plays against a B. But two Type As play far more aggressively, switching their strategies when they think they have the slightest hope of 'screwing the other guy'. And so it is in real life. Suggest to a Type A designer that this season's collection doesn't have much flair, or tell a Type A feature writer that his pieces are becoming predictable and see how they react to you. But for more dramatic results, line them up against other professionals competing for the same commission and see how they react to each other.

Many of those who work on Type A go along with this idea that it only appears when something outside switches it on.

But some of us are not convinced. It may be true that the behaviour needs a trigger, but the committed Type A can find a trigger in almost any situation, at home or on holiday, just as much as at work.

Say the grass needs to be cut. Our Type A householder hates gardening, particularly cutting the lawn. Nonetheless, he won't shrink from his responsibilities. Whatever their faults, Type As are not shirkers. But instead of approaching the job in stages, he will make a huge effort to complete it as a one-stage operation. Like everything else, it has to be finished in the shortest possible time and so it becomes an exercise in frantic activity. The fact that some people can actually enjoy the job is incomprehensible to him. To the Type A the garden is not a source of pleasure; it is a source of challenge.

Then let us follow him on a weekend's vacation (a rare event, but his wife talked him into it). They booked a double room facing the ocean. The room they get is perfect, except that it faces the highway. The receptionist is sorry, but there is nothing he can do. The manager is sorry, but they don't have any other rooms. Within half an hour our Type A weekender has told the staff exactly what he thinks of them and has completely humiliated his wife before setting off to drive the two hundred miles back home.

We can perhaps get some idea of how ingrained the Type A pattern can be by looking at its origins and the way that it develops. Many people ask, 'Is it genetic?' The answer is that parts of the pattern, like tension and hard-driving behaviour, may be inherited. What we actually inherit is probably a particular type of nervous system, wired up in such a way that these features are easily switched on. Some of us may be born with our nervous connections set to react in a Type A direction.

But the greater part of the Type A pattern is undoubtedly learned. It is learned in the home when children are rewarded for being aggressive (parents would say 'assertive'). And it is learned at school when they are rewarded for catching on quickly, performing efficiently and striving to achieve. The Type A child learns what his parents and teachers want him to learn. They shape him for later life and they shape him in their own image. For their part, they see themselves as preparing him to survive and prosper in the hard world outside.

The end result is that speed of performance becomes more important than originality or creativity. Acquisition becomes more important than appreciation, and hostility becomes the automatic response to any event, real or imagined, that he thinks might slow him up or threaten his sense of control. And whatever he may tell you about himself, the fully blown Type A reaches a stage where he derives no satisfaction from any of it. He is locked into a tightening spiral and he may be able to see no way of ever getting off. So he stops looking. He is, in a famous phrase, 'striving without joy'.

Let me prove it to you. The Type A's major goal is to achieve as many things as he can in as short a time as possible, so he constantly finds ways to speed things up. Then he feels the need to occupy the time that he has saved. But everybody's time must eventually become filled by their activities. So the Type A's accelerating lifestyle is inevitably leading him to a point where all his time is accounted for. From the outset, his aims are self-defeating. They are simply destined to bring him face to face with his final frustration, unless he finds some way of getting out. A heart attack is one way, and some Type As I have known became desperate enough almost to welcome it. Then at least the thing could stop.

But what makes Type A behave in this way? Meyer Friedman has suggested that the driving force for the whole complex is simple insecurity.

Obviously most Type A sufferers are not materially or

financially insecure. On the contrary, their efforts result in tangible rewards. Their chronic overworking is something they get paid and promoted for. Their insecurity is much more subtle. It is a basic inability to judge their own worth. Their need for more and more achievement is a constant attempt to prove themselves. It is the Type A's misfortune that he has to demonstrate his worth not to himself, but to those around him. To become convinced of his own value, he needs to have it reflected back at him by those who he feels can appreciate it. But there he puts his head in a noose, because the real Type A won't accept the valuation of his subordinates, even when their views are favourable. Nor will he accept the opinion of his equals. To feel truly valued, he has to catch the attention of his *superiors*. Theirs is the only admiration he will accept. So his whole effort becomes directed at impressing his supervisor, his managing director or his professor, to gain their notice and respect.

If you doubt it, look at what the Type A child is doing in the classroom. He certainly isn't trying to gain the admiration of the other kids. He knows that if he outperforms them they are not going to love him for it. But to impress the teacher, he is prepared to make himself both unhappy and unpopular. And to impress the superiors he meets throughout the rest of his life, he is prepared to go on doing so.

Where are the Type Bs in all this? Many of them are not lacking in ambition either, and they certainly don't hold all the menial jobs. If you look at a cross-section of national leaders, you will find that some of the top positions in business, military and academic life, are occupied by Type Bs. They got there by not compulsively rushing after every deadline in sight nor obsessively trying to reduce each job to a quick mechanical formula. They got there by allowing themselves the time to digest information, to try out different schemes and to experiment. And how did they gain this time? Simply by refusing to be carried along on a tide of hurry, because they did not need to be constantly proving themselves. The Type B carries the measure of his worth inside him. He does not need to have it reflected off others or reinforced by his superiors. Like all of us, he enjoys their admiration, but unlike some of us, he can live without it.

The Type A with his free-floating insecurity is nothing like the hero of all-American enterprises that he first appears to be. His material success gives him progressively less satisfaction as he gets older. A promotion to a higher salary is a measure of how much he is valued, rather than a way of buying the things he wants or needs. Earning and spending give the fully blown Type A little pleasure. He certainly gets things done, but his achievements too lose much of the satisfaction they may once have given him, as they become progressively more mechanical and repetitive – surely reason enough for him to think about making changes. And of course, he's coronary prone. The final irony is that the lifestyle that raises his coronary risk is one that he can't even enjoy.

But he's blinkered as well. He may simply not be capable of looking outside his compulsive behaviour at the possibility of living life differently – until the hospital stay that may follow his first heart attack. There for the first time, in an environment far removed from his business, and sufficiently frightened by the event that brought him there, some Type As might think about changing their ways. The shock was enough for Irving; not so for George.

But as well as change for the better, there is change for the worse. The coronary patient in his mid-forties with a thousand ambitions still unfulfilled may discharge himself from hospital at the earliest moment, to return to them with a desperate vigour, before his precious time runs out. Such men have a death wish. They tell you they don't want to die, but if the risk of death is the trade-off for accomplishing what they want to do, then they accept it, sometimes with a morbid fascination. 'At least it's death with honour,' an A1 friend once told me after his first attack. If Type As had an official song it would have to be 'I Did It My Way'; heroic for the singer, pathetic for anyone listening.

With all this talk of obsession and motivation some psychologists might think that I've gone too far. After all, these ideas about Type A are only 'clinical impressions' – strong feelings that some of the investigators in California have gained about the nature of Type A subjects. And it's certainly true that such observations aren't as firmly based as the WCGS finding that Type A is a coronary risk factor. Even so, I believe that in five or ten years few specialists will doubt them.

Californian researchers have discovered two other basic beliefs that many Type A coronary victims also share. The first is that in today's world, evil often comes out on top. Virtue and goodness go unrewarded. In terms of daily work, that means that your own best efforts usually go unnoticed, while indifferent work by others frequently gets the praise that is yours by right. There's simply no justice.

The other belief is that everything in life – prestige, money, happiness – exists in a limited amount. So everybody has to compete to get his share.

When we put these core beliefs together there emerges a picture of a very unhappy man. He has to be constantly proving himself to his superiors, but he has to do so in a world where there is no automatic guarantee that hard work and good results will be rewarded or even noticed by those whom he wants to impress. The smooth-talking little bastard in the drawing office is as likely to get the credit, even though he contributed hardly anything to the project. In a world with limited resources, the Type A has to hassle constantly to get what is his by right, and to stop his share being stolen by someone else. Is it any wonder that he is hostile?

The extreme Type A's sense of free-floating hostility is his most dangerous feature, not only dangerous for other people, as he would like to think, but even more dangerous for himself. A quarter of a century of experience with Type A coronary patients has shown that the severely hostile person (the man who slams the table while he talks to you in explosive phrases full of obscenity about all the things that irritate him), is a poor treatment prospect. These high-hostile As (maybe a quarter of all Type A coronary victims) are precisely the ones who seem destined for a second heart attack. Finding ways of altering their all-pervasive hostility may be the best contribution to their survival that any counselling can produce.

But it is going to be the most difficult change to make. Type As need their hostility. They need it because they feel themselves surrounded by people who are trying to frustrate them at every turn, and there is nothing like a dose of aggression to keep them all at arm's length. And the need goes even deeper than that.

Some years ago Ray Rosenman together with other investigators who we will meet later, produced a penetrating insight into what the Type A's behaviour is trying to achieve. Their conclusions endorse much of what we now know: 'It is as if these Type As must maintain a high drive and rapid pace in order to gain mastery over their environment.' But what happens when it all seems to be slipping away? 'Impending lack of control is experienced as anxiety-arousing, and leads to task-relevant behaviors designed to assert control.'

Of course, the eventual penalty for this constant vigilance is exhaustion, depression and, when everything goes wrong (and inevitably it sometimes must), a sense of total helplessness. And what do we need to deal with such feelings of failure and weakness? In a word, a burst of aggression. It provides just that surge of arousal that lets the Type A deny any question of being helpless. It allows him to stay on top, where he thinks he belongs, and it doesn't do his image any harm either.

By now we have come close to discovering what Type A really is. It's a series of behaviours designed to gain control and keep it; it's a style of interacting with the outside world; it's a set of private feelings and beliefs. Take your pick. They're all true. They're all facets of the same man.

But they're not the whole of overdrive. Far from it. Overdrive means constantly switching an over-reactive nervous system to 'go'. The Type A's behaviour may increase his risk because it constantly puts him into arousing situations. And if his nervous system's sensitive too, the combination can be lethal. To understand how, we have to look a little more closely both at coronary disease itself and at the way your nervous system works.

3. What Stops the Pump?

If you're lucky, your heart will keep beating about once every second for seventy-odd years. No engineer ever designed a pump remotely as reliable. But all pumps have the same three design features. They need a drive device to force the fluid through. The drive has a control, to give a regular cycle of empty and refill, and the system is hooked up to a fuel supply.

The driving force in the heart is the contraction of the muscle – the *myocardium*. The myocardium has its own built-in pacemaker, but it also receives electrical impulses from the nerve supply connecting it with the brain. Actually there are two nerve networks because the heart needs a variable speed. It has to be able to provide blood either fast or slowly, depending on the body's constantly changing demands.

The nerve supply acting as the accelerator is called the *sympathetic* system. Sympathetic impulses cause the heart to speed up and increase the force of each myocardial contraction so that more blood is pumped every second. Anyone who has ever been angry or excited; run round a track or skied down a slope; or sat in a sauna bath, has felt the sympathetic nerves driving his heart in response to the emotion, exercise or heat.

The heart's decelerator (sometimes even its brake) is known as the *parasympathetic* system. When parasympathetic messages reach the myocardium from the brain, the heart rate falls and the pump pressure drops. Anyone who has had to suffer a pain they could not escape (the dentist's drill), or been nauseated by scenes of cruelty (ovens in Belsen, napalm in Vietnam), has felt the influence of the parasympathetic nerves on his heart. But then, so too has anyone who has felt the relief of some major ordeal being over (the blood tests are negative). These impulses reach your heart through one of the body's major nerves – the *vagus*. So physicians often use a shorthand. Instead of talking about the parasympathetic system, they simply talk about *vagal effects*.

Most of the time the vagus is in control. When you are sitting or lying, your pulse rate stays fairly constant and the amount of blood leaving your heart every minute (your *cardiac output*) is steady. When your pulse starts to increase, it does so first because the vagal influence gets weaker; the brake is taken off. Only then does the sympathetic system take over. The accelerator is pressed to serve an extra demand on the pump. Unfortunately, many of us go around pressing the accelerator for much of the day. The dedicated overdriver lives much of his waking life that way. The long-term result may be pump failure, often with a clogged-up fuel pipe, because the heart's fuel supply is the weakest feature in its design.

Every muscle needs oxygen and that oxygen comes from the blood. But though the heart pumps out a gallon a minute, little of the oxygen dissolved in its blood-filled chambers reaches the heart muscle itself. Oxygen is for export, and the heart's own oxygen has to be re-imported. With each contraction, the main pumping chamber forces blood into the body's largest artery – the *aorta*. From the aorta arise the arteries that carry blood to all other organs, except the lungs, which have a separate supply. And the very first branches coming off the aorta are the two arteries that supply blood to the myocardium. One divides into two soon after it reaches the heart, and so the myocardium gets its blood from three vital vessels, vital because its working depends entirely on their ability to provide it with fuel.

The three arteries that lie on the heart's outer surface were thought by the early anatomists to surround it like a crown (though I have never been able to see the resemblance myself). The Latin word for crown is *corona*, and so they came to be known as the *coronary arteries*. Latin or not, there can be few of us who have never heard of coronary artery disease, a complaint that medical men abbreviate to CAD. They have another abbreviation too – CHD – for coronary heart disease. The two sound similar enough, but the difference between them is all-important.

No one who has seen the literature put out by, say, the World Health Organization, the National Institutes of Health or the American Heart Association, and recycled in a thousand magazines, can doubt that diseased coronary arteries are extremely common in Western countries. There are probably more men over thirty-five in Britain and America with partly blocked arteries than without. Post-mortems carried out on people dying from all causes, suggest that the number of living Americans with CAD is as high as a hundred million. Sometimes it was difficult to know how the victims survived for as long as they did.

And CAD isn't confined to the elderly, or even the middle-aged. In the mid-1950s many physicians were surprised by a report on the coronary arteries of soldiers who had died in combat in Korea. After examining a group of three hundred of them, the pathologists reported 'some gross evidence of coronary disease' in three out of four. Their average age was slightly over twenty-two. And while combat casualties in Vietnam some fifteen years later were in rather better shape, half of them also had some coronary blockage.

The most disturbing fact about CAD is that you can have it for years without knowing. Often it causes no distress, and even an electrocardiogram in the doctor's surgery may not detect it. But the moment that it starts to cause trouble, the situation changes. When the coronary arteries fail, it is the heart that suffers. And the instant your heart discovers its arteries aren't working properly is the instant we stop talking about CAD and start talking about CHD instead.

Coronary heart disease can show itself in at least three different ways. The first is *angina pectoris*, Latin again, literally meaning a pain in the breast. The pain is usually felt in the middle of the chest underneath the breast bone (not two inches below the left nipple, where many hypochondriacs imagine their hearts to be). It may spread across the shoulder, down the arm or up into the jaw. When severe, it has been described as 'like being in a vice'. The chest is tight and the sufferer often has to fight for his breath. He may sweat and shiver at the same time.

Fortunately, angina isn't always so severe. Some sufferers go for years having only mild attacks with weeks or months in between. But for others the attacks get more frequent as time goes by. They are nearly always brought on either by exertion (running upstairs, pushing the car, shovelling snow) or by emotion (screaming at the kids to get out of the bathroom, or promising yourself that the very next time that the supervisor insults you, you'll tell him exactly where to put his job). The pain can usually be relieved by taking nitroglycerine, better known perhaps as an explosive, and more recent drugs have also been developed to deal with it.

Coronary death is the second way in which CHD can show itself. Often it too follows exertion or emotion. Sometimes, though not always, it is preceded by warning attacks of angina. The victim collapses and dies within hours, sometimes minutes. Coroners may distinguish between the first type of death which they call 'sudden', and the second, in which the deceased's departure is described as 'instantaneous'.

What actually kills him? There are several possibilities. The first is a sudden surge of vagal impulses that slows his heart down so much that it stops beating altogether. And what causes the surge? Bad news or an inescapable emotional shock have both been known to do it.

But the human heart takes some stopping and perhaps only one in five sudden deaths is caused in this way. More often it results from a surge, not of vagal, but of sympathetic impulses. The heart receives volleys of electrical signals, each one making it contract, but they are all out of phase. They don't arrive in any orderly pattern. So the different parts of the myocardium contract at random. The heart looks like 'a can of writhing worms'. This random contraction is known as *fibrillation*. It overrides the regular pattern and stops any blood from being pumped at all. Unless the normal rhythm is restored very quickly by a controlled, synchronized electric shock (defibrillation) death will result as the body, and particularly the brain and the heart itself, have their oxygen cut off.

And what causes the massive surge in sympathetic traffic? It is often impossible to say. But there have been enough sudden deaths involving exertion or emotion, or worse still, both of them together, for us to be quite sure that either of them can do it. The salesman who can't find a taxi and runs two blocks with his order books to clinch a sale is taking the same risk as the middle-aged lawyer who punishes himself getting his marathon time inside three hours, just to show his son's friends he can do it. Both are risking fibrillation. If they collapse more than a few minutes away from a defibrillator (and the vast majority do) their chances of survival are remote.

The third type of CHD is the one that people seem to know most about – *myocardial infarction* or MI. We know, for example, that it is an attack from which you may stand some chance of recovery. It is often called a 'coronary thrombosis' and many of us have read that it can be caused by a clot in one of the coronary arteries cutting off the blood supply to some particular region of the heart. If a vital region of the myocardium is affected – if, for example, one of the pacemaker areas is destroyed – then the attack will probably be fatal. If not, the victim may survive, at least if he gets to hospital quickly enough.

So far so good. But the debit side is chilling. You may be dead within a matter of minutes. Of a thousand fatal infarctions in Belfast, (one of the first cities to introduce mobile coronary care in the 1960s) one man in four and one woman in five were dead within a quarter of an hour. The average survival time for all the male victims was only three and a half hours and it is not surprising that six out of ten died without seeing the inside of a hospital.

The cause of death after infarction is usually fibrillation, or some serious disorganization of the heart's normal rhythm, a so-called *fatal arrhythmia*. But if you are carrying a piece of dead or dying muscle around in your heart, then arrhythmias can recur more or less any time. So a patient who survives the initial attack through prompt hospital care still has a greatly increased risk of a second. According to one estimate, he is about thirty times more likely to die in the first year than a healthy man of the same age. The risk falls with time, so that after ten years the two men's odds are similar. But a decade is a long time to be apprehensive. The number of deaths from infarction have fallen in the last ten years in the USA (though not, it seems, in Britain), but even today, one patient in every five never leaves the hospital alive, and few of those who do go home ever return to a completely normal lifestyle.

Recently it has also been discovered that the coronary arteries in some susceptible people may close up spontaneously, even though they are not blocked. Rather than a furred-up fuel pipe, you can think of the pipe being gripped by pliers. After seconds or minutes the spasm relaxes and blood flows to the myocardium again. But the heart experiences the oxygen starvation as a period of pain, anginal pain. And in some cases the spasm might prove fatal. It may be some consolation to know that you would be exceptional if this happened to you, though of course if you're over thirty-five and male, you would be exceptional to have coronary arteries with no blockage already.

But the block has to be rather large before it starts to make its presence felt, and sometimes there are years of delay before CAD becomes CHD. Having a coronary artery even half blocked at some point may not affect the blood flow seriously enough to cause angina. As much as three-quarters has to be obstructed before we start to feel the effects.

Whether it kills us depends on whether we put excessive demands on our heart muscle, demands that the restricted blood supply cannot meet. Instantaneous death during exertion seems to be an extreme case of supply falling behind demand. The exercise increases the heart's need for oxygen, but the coronary blockage stops it from getting there. Now that procedures for measuring coronary artery obstruction are fairly routine, it might become possible to detect individuals with a particularly high risk of instantaneous death and warn them in advance. Whether they heed the warning is another issue.

But the question of when CAD becomes fatal may also depend on whether the blood inside the artery forms a clot. More than eight out of ten heart patients who died within hours (rather than minutes) in one Californian study had coronary thromboses, and many other post-mortems have found the same. In these cases it seems the combination of a thickened arterial wall *plus* the extra blockage of a clot resulted in their sudden departure. The blockage doesn't even have to cause an infarction (though it may). If the blood supply is restricted enough, the heart may still go into fibrillation, just as it does with instantaneous death.

Hardening and narrowing of the arteries occurs when their

linings become thickened with a grey, greasy-looking material called *atheroma*. When the process is progressive, we call it *atherosclerosis*.

The sequence of events seems to be like this. Only a delicate layer of cells lines the artery, to separate the arterial wall with its muscle fibres on one side, from the blood in the channel on the other. This lining may become damaged, perhaps because high blood pressure puts an excessive strain on the vessel wall, or because some of the poisonous ingredients in cigarette smoke get into the blood stream and affect the arterial cells. Once the lining is breached, chemical substances from the blood, particularly cholesterol, can get inside. Cholesterol is thought to make the muscle cells of the arterial wall multiply and produce a protein substance called *collagen*. As a result of these changes, the lining of the artery swells out into the central channel. It forms a thick cushion packed with cholesterol, muscle cells and collagen, a constricting hump known as a *plaque*.

As long as the plaque remains intact it doesn't present any immediate threat to life. You simply have CAD. But as it gets bigger, it may start to break up inside, like an abscess. When this happens, the surface layer of cells that has been covering it and separating it from the circulating blood all this time breaks up too. Blood gets into the plaque. Within the blood are many millions of tiny platelets, cells much smaller than red corpuscles, whose purpose it is to settle in any wounded tissue, clump together, and clot. This is the first stage in any tissue repair and without it we would all bleed to death. The platelets gather in the dissolving plaque, trying to close up the gap that its breakdown has made in the arterial wall. But the plaque has lots of collagen, which makes blood clots form fast and large. Once the platelets contact the collagen the clot can start to increase out of control. It may block the already restricted channel, cutting off the blood supply to the heart completely.

If the blockage is small or short-lived, or if it occurs in a minor artery, then any resulting infarction may go almost unnoticed. Doctors talk about 'silent infarction', attacks so minor that the sufferer took them for indigestion – Irving's 'heartburn'. But if the blockage remains and if the other coronary vessels can't make up the shortfall, then the resulting heart attack may be massive and fatal – George's second attack.

That at least is one scenario for coronary thrombosis. Other specialists have other views. Some think that the clot forms first. Others believe that the platelets actually produce the plaque. But whatever the details, we will only understand the process properly when we know what damages the arterial lining, what makes plaques grow and develop, what makes platelets sticky and what causes the heart, on occasions, to demand more oxygen than its arteries can supply.

Overdrive is part of the answer – and an important part. By living the way they do, overdrivers may speed up the blockage of their coronary arteries. Certainly as a result of their behaviour they increase the stickiness of their blood platelets, disturb their heart's normal rhythm, and risk directly damaging their myocardium. The overdriver constantly tips the balance of his nervous system towards the sympathetic side and sympathetic arousal has far-reaching effects.

And of course, he makes it so much worse if he smokes. Today only a few die-hards seriously question the fact that cigarettes kill people. When a group of British doctors gave up smoking, their risks of a fatal heart attack were halved in five years. When Californian physicians did the same, their cancer and heart disease rates came down too.

What risks are we talking about? The biggest ever assessment of coronary risk factors was the US Pooling Project which we will look at in more detail later. This

Project found that men smoking a pack of cigarettes a day (and most smokers do) had two and a half times more chance of coronary disease than non-smokers. Cigar and pipe smokers didn't seem to have a greater risk at all, but there weren't that many of them. The Project team admitted that a larger study would be necessary to decide whether pipe and cigar risks really were as low as they seemed, and more recent figures suggest that they're not.

The Pooling Project was only concerned with heart disease, but tobacco can kill you in other ways as well. At least a quarter of all cancer deaths in American men and 5–10 per cent of those in women are directly due to smoking. Recently the deaths of half a million men in the United States were related to their smoking habits. The difference in life expectancy at the age of thirty-five between those who never smoked and those smoking forty a day was nearly eight years. Of America's fifty million smokers, nearly half are women, and three out of four infarctions in women under forty-five would be prevented if they simply didn't smoke.

Why do cigarettes produce such a heart disease risk, to say nothing of the risks of cancer? First, the carbon monoxide in the smoke stops red blood cells from carrying as much oxygen as they otherwise would, so it cuts down the oxygen supply to the heart muscle. At the same time, the nicotine that smokers do it all for releases a substance called noradrenaline, one of the stimulants of the sympathetic nervous system, which increases both your heart rate and blood pressure. So the pump has to work harder on a lower grade fuel. Noradrenaline may disturb the rhythm of the already struggling pump and even damage the myocardium itself. And that's not all. Smoking increases the stickiness of the blood platelets, so that thrombosis is more likely. At the same time, by damaging the arterial wall, it may let platelets and cholesterol get inside and so help stimulate the formation of atheroma. And by now we know that fatal equation:

atheroma plus thrombosis equals heart attack.

Cigarettes also make arteries close down in other parts of your body. The legs usually go first. As the arterial disease progresses, walking becomes painful, then impossible, and in some cases surgery is the only answer. Yet the committed smoker still carries on, driven by a real addiction. Some years ago a documentary television crew filmed a three-pack-a-day man in his home. The camera caught him in close up, devouring the last half inch of a cigarette. No, he told the earnest young interviewer, he wasn't prepared to give up, 'Not even after what the doctors told me. Not even after the operations.'

'Operations?'

The camera panned down to the place where his legs should have been. His arterial disease had gone so far that both of them had been amputated at the knee. But 'Oh yes,' he said, 'I really do enjoy a cigarette.'

4. Effort, Distress and Your Adrenals

How are workers who spend all day sorting components or operating presses different from foresters or blacksmiths? Not only do they work inside, in one position, at a job that gives them little exercise, but, more important, they have higher rates of myocardial infarction. They also have higher infarction rates than doctors or lawyers, janitors or nightwatchmen. Indeed production-line workers have more heart disease than people in most other types of job. There seems to be something about machine-paced work that damages their health.

The question is what? You may still hear some of those who talk about 'executive's disease' suggesting that it is the white-collar workers, particularly the managers, whose health suffers most as a result of their jobs. But the idea is thirty years out of date. David Jenkins has put the situation rather well: 'Early in the process of industrial development in a nation, individuals with higher education and those with prestigious occupations tend to have higher rates of coronary heart disease. As the industrial revolution proceeds, it has been the general pattern for the tide of the greatest risk to flow downwards and begin accumulating in the lower social levels.'

This change started to show itself in the 1950s. A 1958 examination of over a thousand American executives reported 'surprisingly' (their own word) that high blood pressure (hypertension) was no more frequent than it was among non-executives, and that cardiovascular disease was actually lower. They suggested that only the healthiest might get to the top, or perhaps the executives learned to judge the amount of 'occupational stress' that they could stand. Another study of some six hundred Du Pont employees who had heart attacks in the mid-1950s found that the highest salary earners had only half the infarction rate of the lowest. The team reporting the finding made what for the time was a novel suggestion: 'Persons occupying higher managerial positions may derive a great deal of satisfaction from the demands of their job, while those at lower levels and with a minimum of responsibility may suffer from feelings of resentment and frustration due to the lack of personal fulfilment and their relatively low position on the socio-economic scale.'

The investigation that more or less clinched the matter (and there have been many since) was a now famous five-year study of 270,000 employees of the Bell Telephone Company. Men who reached the highest managerial levels had no more coronary disease than those lower down. Nor was there evidence of any added coronary risk resulting from a high level of job responsibility or frequent promotion.

All this is not to say that managers don't die from heart disease – they do. Nor does it mean that they don't have special problems of their own. After all, the Type A pattern is found more among those with high-status jobs. What it does mean is that 'executive's disease' is a complicated problem. And looking at illness among managers has given us a clearer understanding of the health hazards faced by machine-minders as well. The factors that influence the executive's health – like workload, satisfaction and responsibility – are the same for any worker doing any job. Where jobs differ is in the balance between them.

In 1968, 1500 Swedish working men were interviewed about their jobs. They were asked whether the work was hectic and psychologically demanding. The investigators were also interested in a second dimension. They wanted to know whether the worker could exercise much discretion over what he was doing, and whether the job allowed him very much personal freedom. These factors are difficult to define, but the survey team settled for a rough estimate.

An example of work with very low discretion was a repetitive job that needed only a minimum level of education. A non-repetitive job, that took more than four years' extra education to be able to do it at all, was described as one with high discretion. Personal freedom was even more difficult to assess, but if workers could make at least one private phone call during working hours, see a private visitor for ten minutes and leave the job for half an hour of private errands without having to tell their supervisor, then they were thought to have a high level of freedom. Those who could do none of these things had only a low level.

The men were followed up to see whether any coronary symptoms appeared during the five or six years after the interview. Those who died were compared with survivors who resembled them closely at the start of the survey, to see whether any job differences would emerge between the living and the dead. And they did.

Having a hectic and psychologically demanding job increased the risk of developing symptoms of CHD, such as chest pain and shortness of breath. Even worse, it went with an actual increase in deaths from coronary disease and stroke. And for the majority of workers in the survey (and in the country) with only a minimum level of education, having little personal freedom on the job also carried an increased risk of death. Such differences could not be explained away by smoking or overweight. When these other risk factors were controlled for, as they were in the Western Collaborative Group Study, the increased job risk still remained.

The focus of attention then swung to the United States.

The same research team (a group that included Dr Robert A. Karasek, of Columbia University, New York, and Dr Töres Theorell, who had been responsible for generating much of the original Swedish data) made use of two large-scale American health surveys, each involving some two thousand workers. The workers had been given a full examination, including a medical history, chest X-ray, and electrocardiogram, so it was possible to decide how many of them were suffering from the symptoms of a past myocardial infarction. Both surveys also had details of the men's occupations, so that it was possible to match their job to their disease pattern.

But how to assess the job itself – its physical and psychological demands, the opportunity to make decisions and so on? Fortunately, the US Department of Labor had already conducted other studies in which members of the work force in over two hundred different occupations had described their jobs in enough detail to estimate, for each job description, just how psychologically demanding it was and how much freedom the worker had to make his own decisions.

Karasek and his team were the first to admit that such descriptions can only be approximate. After all, two men may both describe themselves as bakers, but one 'may be rolling artistic croissants in a French pastry shop; the other working in a mass-production bread-loaf bakery'. And the sort of investigation that they could perform, being able to link infarction to the type of job at only one moment in time, could never be as revealing as a long-term follow-up study like Framingham or the WCGS.

Even so, their results were very interesting. They discovered four basic types of occupation. In 'high strain' jobs, demands are high but control is low. This applies to many machine-paced and time-structured jobs, like the assemblers and press-operators we started with. Then came what they called 'active' jobs, where demands are also high, but so too is the control that you can exert over them. Doctors, lawyers and many managers come into this category. Among the 'low strain' group, with a combination of low demands and high control, they included research scientists and conservationists. And finally, in the so-called 'passive' group, we have workers with low control, but low demands on them as well, like the janitors and watchmen we also met at the beginning.

The research team had already discovered that the highest levels of psychological strain – sleep problems, depression, job dissatisfaction and so on – were found among workers in high strain jobs. With this survey they found a clear increase in myocardial infarction among workers in high strain occupations as well. Low decision latitude was related to infarction in both surveys. Indeed, after age (obviously, older people have more susceptibility to disease), having little ability to make decisions on the job was the *strongest* risk factor for MI, stronger even than raised cholesterol. Mentally demanding work also went with infarction, but it didn't seem to be as big a risk. Overall, the greatest risk of heart attacks occurred among those carrying a high psychological workload but with little opportunity to make their own decisions.

We can best understand how these work-related factors translate into disease by considering the research carried out by a second Swedish group, this one led by Dr Marianne Frankenhaeuser, who is currently Professor of Psychology in the University of Stockholm. David Jenkins once defined work overload as: 'a chronic demand for rapid, precise behaviors with sustained vigilance under high pressure, and the threat of trouble if errors occur'. Marianne Frankenhaeuser's team have examined what that means in practice.

They looked initially at Swedish saw-mill workers, men

faced with particular work pressures. Those who actually sawed the timber had to judge continually what they were doing and how best to do it. Mistakes could be expensive as well as dangerous. But they also had to keep up with the machine, and just to do that required nearly all their attention. The work cycle was amazingly short. From the arrival of the log to the finished cutting might take only ten seconds. The cutters were all skilled men, well able to make expert judgements, but they had to work at such a speed that they had little chance to use their skills properly. Naturally enough, they felt an almost continuous sense of frustration. Add to that the fact that they had to work in the same position for much of the shift, that the noise in the saw-house stopped any normal conversation, and that they were paid piece-work rates, and you have a perfect example of a high strain job.

Their health records showed it. Compared with men working elsewhere in the same mills, those in the saw-house were more tired, tense and anxious. They took more sick leave and had more frequent cardiovascular and nervous disorders.

To the Swedish investigators, it seemed that even more than their total workload, the key factor leading to their discomfort and illness was the lack of control over their jobs. This put them into a constant state of arousal – in fact over-arousal. They were aroused far beyond the levels at which they could function best.

One way to study arousal is to look at the body's production of two biochemicals, *adrenaline* and *noradrenaline*, both of which put your heart rate and blood pressure up. They can be measured either in the blood or (more conveniently, if less accurately) in samples of urine. The Swedish team collected urine samples from the saw-house men at 6 a.m. when they arrived for work, and at various times during the working day. For comparison, samples were collected from the same men at the same times but on their rest days when they were staying at home. Both chemicals were also measured in a group of repair and maintenance men who didn't have to keep up with the machine, and who generally had a lot more freedom over the speed and rhythm of their work.

At most times in their working day, both adrenaline and noradrenaline were higher in the saw operators than in the maintenance men. They were more aroused for more of the time. The two groups also showed different patterns. For the repair men, both substances reached a peak after a couple of hours' work, then started to fall again. But for the saw-men they both went on increasing through the afternoon, to reach peak levels when the day was actually over. So they took the effects of a hectic work shift home with them. And this fits with the men's own description of being tense and exhausted, sometimes too tired even to speak to their wife or children for hours after they got back home.

This 'hangover' also occurs in jobs that are much less demanding than spending eight hours behind a circular saw. When women invoice clerks in the Swedish National Telecommunications Administration were paid piece-work rates instead of their usual weekly wage for an experimental period, their work output certainly increased. But so did their feelings of rush, fatigue and discomfort. On days when they were paid piece rates, their adrenalines were up by a half and their noradrenalines by a quarter. Confectionery workers in Italy showed two- to fivefold rises when they were transferred from fixed wages to piece rates.

A more common way of making extra money is to keep the same wage level but to volunteer for overtime. A group of Swedish women insurance clerks were invited to do just that – to work seventy-two hours' overtime over a period of six weeks. They could choose when to put in the extra hours, and most of them opted for the weekends. When they were asked how it was affecting them, many said that they felt tired and irritable and some said that their hearts were beating faster, even at home. Urine samples showed that their adrenaline levels were raised right through the overtime period, both during the day and in the evenings. Since most of them did their household chores at weekends, they felt a divided loyalty between the job and the house that was probably important in putting their adrenalines up.

And just getting to work can do something similar. Anyone who has to commute into the city on a train that is dirty, late and overcrowded is used to the signals from his body telling his brain that the trip is doing neither of them any good. The basis of these signals (the quick and heavy heartbeat, the difficulty in concentrating and the strong desire to be somewhere else) was examined during the petrol shortage in 1974, when the number of Swedish commuters increased by 10 per cent. That doesn't seem much (until you're on the train) but travellers' estimates of crowding are badly biased. An actual threefold increase of people in a railway carriage is estimated as a tenfold rise by the passengers themselves. So 10 per cent was quite enough to disturb their equilibrium.

Uncrowded commuting caused adrenaline to increase by 20 per cent over the 'baseline' level that the same passengers had on days when they didn't travel. But an extra load of one body in ten gave them an adrenaline rise of 60 per cent. And they weren't strap-hanging for twenty miles either. Everyone got a seat. What they didn't get was the freedom to choose which seat or to choose the people they sat with. Passengers who got on the train first had lower adrenalines than those who got on midway. Firstcomers had more choice and more control.

And indeed, what all these hassling situations have in common is precisely that – a struggle for control. The worker on the circular saw has a constant struggle over the way the job has to be done. He could do it better, but the machine moves too fast to let him. The piece-rate worker struggles to increase her output and boost her pay packet. The over-time worker struggles with the conflicting demands of her job and her home. The commuter struggles to sit where he wants.

They are all actively trying to achieve something, and to cope with the situation they find themselves in. So, to use the psychologist's jargon, they are all engaged in 'active coping'. One result of active coping is a rise in *catecholamines* – a word used to describe both adrenaline and noradrenaline together. But different kinds of coping seem to produce different responses.

Many research groups have tried to discover just what sort of threat or challenge causes an adrenaline rise, or what kind of stimulus puts your noradrenaline up. At one time it was thought that adrenaline goes up when you're afraid, noradrenaline when you're angry. But this turned out to be too simple. It now seems more likely that adrenaline increases during any type of emotional arousal. So it goes up in situations that you find strange or unpredictable, where you are aroused and waiting for something to happen. But such anticipation often does have an element of fear about it – hence the original theory.

Noradrenaline doesn't seem to be linked very closely to emotion, though it does often rise when we get angry. It responds more strongly to physical activity. So running or lifting weights puts noradrenaline levels up. But in real life there aren't many situations that produce pure emotion or pure activity. When you anticipate something unpleasant you may be active and agitated. You switch on both systems. And when you exercise hard it hurts, but it also lifts your mood. You get an emotional response, often a feeling of power quite close to anger. Again, you turn both systems on.

Most of the situations that cause catecholamines to rise call for effort. You are engaged, involved, trying to achieve something or trying to cope with an event that is forcing itself on your attention.

Let's look at a few.

Driving a car is something that most of us do every day, and yet a two-hour drive, even in your own car in ordinary traffic, will practically double the catecholamines excreted in your urine. At least, if you're a man it will – women seem less reactive. Some racing drivers have shown tenfold increases following a competition. The majority of the rise was noradrenaline, which may confirm the link with anger. Driving at this level is an aggressive sport. But it's physically taxing too, and much of the increase might simply be due to the continuous effort of keeping a big car on the track.

Talking to groups of people is something else that most of us have to do occasionally. All of us feel nervous about it, especially if the outcome is important for our job or our self-image. Whether it's the salesman presenting to a group of clients ('We're sure this is the main-frame for your business'); the high school teacher with a group of students ('I know how you feel, believe me') or the young doctor explaining his diagnosis to his superiors ('Yes sir, I did consider that possibility'), the body's reaction is the same – a catecholamine surge.

The effect has been looked at closely in a group of young doctors at the Massachusetts General Hospital in Boston. They volunteered to have blood samples taken while they were describing their patients' progress to their senior colleagues. By putting a thin tube into an arm vein and linking it to a small pump, it was possible to collect blood samples continuously as the doctors went about their everyday activities. Samples were taken soon after the line was inserted, to give a measure of normal 'baseline' levels, and again during the first minute of their address. Their adrenalines reached twice the baseline value when they started talking. Noradrenaline went up too, though not so much.

To confirm that noradrenaline responds better to exertion, the same volunteers were asked to run up and down twenty flights of stairs. Blood samples taken during the exercise showed a slight rise in adrenaline, but a threefold noradrenaline increase. At least, it was threefold on average. Some volunteers showed twice that much. These individual differences are something we meet time and time again when we look at the reactions of different people.

Before young doctors get to treat patients at all they have to take a long series of examinations. Since everything depends on passing, their responses under exam conditions represent active coping at its sharpest. Medical students in Britain had their chemical reactions examined during a fifteen-minute oral examination in anatomy. Adrenaline levels more than doubled, and noradrenaline rose by 70 per cent. Again though, there was a wide spread of results, and some of these young men reacted far beyond the average.

A six-hour matriculation exam was also used in Finland to study catecholamine changes in a group of eighteen-year-old high school students. For most of them, both adrenaline and noradrenaline increased in response to this important challenge – getting a job might depend on it. The rises were less in the girls than the boys but there was no difference (among students who had really tried) in the results that they achieved. It simply seems that the girls responded to the challenge in a more 'economical' way.

The same sex differences can be seen at an even younger age. Another Scandinavian group looked at the reactions of thirteen-year-olds who were given a mental arithmetic test and told that they really had to do well. Urine samples collected after the test meant that the catecholamines excreted during the exam could be measured. Again, the rises were more marked for boys than for girls, but a second difference also became clear. By looking at the children's normal grades and talking to their teachers, it was possible to pick out a group of boys best described as 'over-achievers'. Catecholamine levels among these over-achievers were higher than for any of the others.

Sounds familiar – the over-achieving Type A child trying to impress his teacher and please his parents? The study didn't actually measure Type A but its authors noticed that the boys fell into two groups. Some were 'neurotic' over-achievers, who had other people's demands thrust upon them. But there were others who had their *own* motivation to do well and simply felt more secure in achievement-oriented situations. If they're like that at thirteen, it's hardly surprising that they're difficult to save from themselves when they become high coronary risks twenty years later.

Driving, public speaking and being examined cause both of the catecholamines to rise. But physicians have tried for a long time to find behaviours that stimulate just one or the other. The nearest thing to a pure response seems to result from smoking. Dr Malcolm Carruthers, now at the Maudsley Hospital in London, wasn't the first to discover this fact, but he did show what happens if you smoke three cigarettes, one after the other. Levels of adrenaline in your blood stream hardly change at all. But noradrenaline goes up sharply. And it goes up most after smoking cigarettes with a high nicotine content. The nicotine stimulus is obviously what smokers are going for, but it seems that nicotine might only be the trigger. The bullet is noradrenaline. What the smoker is trying to do without realizing it, is to boost his noradrenaline level.

Why? Because, as Carruthers and other research workers have suggested, stimulating the brain with noradrenaline might be the ultimate fix – the 'final common pathway' for many forms of pleasure.

The idea goes back to the mid-1950s when it was found that rats with electrodes placed in a particular region of their brain would rather spend their time pressing a lever to give themselves electrical stimulation than get involved in any more obviously pleasurable activity, like eating or mating. Clearly, the stimulation must be intensely pleasurable in itself. Later research suggested that the electric current was actually releasing noradrenaline, which then stimulated particular 'pleasure centres' inside the brain. And from there it was only a short step to imagine that any pleasurable human behaviour might be doing the same thing – releasing noradrenaline to switch on the brain activity that we recognize as pleasure.

This isn't the place to ask whether pleasure centres really exist, and if they do, what turns them on. Suffice it to say that most specialists don't think that pleasure is simply a belt of noradrenaline released inside the brain. The whole system seems much more complicated and may involve the more recently discovered 'endorphins', natural substances with morphine-like effects. Even so, the idea shouldn't be scrapped. It may be simple but some facts fit it very well. What about the 'runner's high', the feeling of near ecstasy that some people get ten miles or so into a run? We know that running releases noradrenaline. How ironic if the exercise addiction had the same basis as the tobacco craving.

And what gives the workaholic his compulsion? The successful middle-aged Type A doesn't have to work so hard. He doesn't really choose to either. It has simply become a habit, a deeply ingrained addictive habit that he doesn't know how to break. When he tries, for a week, or a weekend, perhaps even for a day, he gets the withdrawal symptoms that send him running back to the office. Could it be that like the pack-a-day smoker, he too is simply addicted? Any overdriver will tell you that to be successful you have to keep the adrenaline flowing. Perhaps he is describing his compulsion better than he knows. He's simply got his catecholamines mixed up.

Adrenaline and noradrenaline are both released by the

sympathetic nervous system, the heart's accelerator that we met in the last chapter, though the two originate in different places. Noradrenaline is found in the nerves that connect the brain with the heart and blood vessels. In response to an electrical brain impulse, a small package of noradrenaline is released from the nerve ending to stimulate the heart. And the impulses pass in abundance when you are called upon to make a particular physical effort.

Adrenaline, by contrast, comes from the adrenals, two small glands which lie just above your kidneys. Unlike noradrenaline, which is released directly on to its target tissue, adrenaline is a hormone. It is secreted into the blood stream and it circulates round the body. Its secretion is suddenly boosted by a whole range of conditions – fear or environmental overload among them.

Sympathetic arousal usually involves both catecholamines, and certainly when we are very aroused we feel the effects of both. They produce a series of bodily changes that prepare us to meet a physical or emotional challenge. Our heart rate and the force of our heart beat increase, so that more blood is pumped every second. Blood is shunted away from regions where it is not immediately required, like the skin and intestines, into the blood vessels that supply our major muscles, particularly in the arms and legs. These vessels dilate and the increased blood flow brings extra oxygen and fuel to prepare the muscle for action.

The whole system has been developed over a long period of evolution, and our stone-age forebears inherited it from their primate ancestors. It prepared them either to face the challenge (usually from an animal, or from some other human beings) or else run away from it. So medical textbooks for half a century have described it as the 'fight-or-flight' reaction. Those of our ancestors who were able to produce the response as soon as the challenge appeared would have an advantage over the others. Rather than being taken by surprise and laying themselves open, they would be psyched up in anticipation, with hearts pumping and muscles ready for action.

Today we still go through exactly the same responses when we are challenged. The difference is that, muggings aside, today's challenges usually threaten our economic status, our social position or our self-esteem, rather than our lives or physical well-being. And many of us still retain the ability to respond in anticipation of trouble. Indeed, we anticipate and respond to many situations that never actually develop.

So here we are, stuck with a relic of palaeolithic times. Moderate arousal is essential for our continued survival and well-being. But there are few situations that urban man has to face today that call for a massive physical effort or a full-scale rage reaction. Sitting in traffic or making a sales pitch are certainly not among them, and yet both can produce catecholamine surges.

It's not just that such responses are inappropriate. They're positively dangerous. Yet many of us make them, many times a day. Those who do, I have called overdrivers. Regularly over-arousing your sympathetic system is a definition of the overdriver's way of life.

And the consequences are frightening. Take, for example, the rise in blood pressure that results from a massive anger reaction. We know that increased blood pressure can damage the delicate arterial lining, leading to tears that may become sites for atheroma. The more often we drive our blood pressure up (or let someone else do it for us) the more often we risk such an injury. Some specialists even believe that permanently raised blood pressure, or hypertension, may arise as a result of these pressure jags. Among the best known is Dr Stevo Julius of Michigan University, who has said quite specifically that: 'Sympathetic nervous system overactivity, present in some patients with borderline hypertension, may lead to the later development of established hypertension.'

He may be right, but we don't need to go so far. Just letting it rise and fall a dozen or more times a day, may be quite enough to accelerate your atheroma, even though your baseline pressure is hardly raised.

Increased blood pressure may start a plaque, but a different disturbance makes it grow. If cholesterol gets into the damaged artery it can cause an increase in the number of muscle cells in the arterial wall. So any increase in cholesterol in the blood may hasten the growth of a plaque. Your sympathetic system can make that happen too.

Catecholamines provide energy for the working muscles. During arousal, most of the energy comes in the form of fats. Your fatty tissues are broken down to produce substances known as free fatty acids and triglycerides, which circulate in the blood and act as energy sources. But they're not only produced as part of muscular fight-or-flight. Anger releases them as well, and so do hassle and distress.

For example, one group of Swedish volunteers were asked to spend two hours sorting ball-bearings – not an easy task, because they were all much the same size. To make it more like real-life work, they also had to endure loud industrial noise and flashing lights, and they had to work under time pressure, so that they were constantly hurrying the job. Not surprisingly, they described themselves as 'moderately aroused' by all this, and their urinary adrenalines and noradrenalines both went up. So too did the free fatty acids and triglycerides in their blood. During active physical work, these substances get used up. But when we just have to sit there, they are not broken down nearly as fast. Through a complicated series of changes, triglycerides may help to carry cholesterol into the walls of your arteries. So, sympathetic arousal helps plaques to grow. The free fatty acids are also a hazard, because they can disturb the heart's normal rhythm.

Catecholamines can also cause arrhythmias, for example, when we have to endure distressing situations, as many of us know from experience. These disturbed rhythms have been studied in experimental animals. It is possible to produce fibrillation in dogs by applying a small voltage to their heart at a particular moment during the heart beat (the dogs are then treated with a defibrillator and they make a complete recovery). When such a shock is given in the rather unfriendly environment of the laboratory, a smaller voltage is needed to disturb the rhythm than when the dogs are in their own cages. In other words, the threshold for fibrillation is lowered by exposing them to distress or discomfort. And this is just as true for us .

Although the ability to turn on the fight-or-flight reaction in a matter of seconds may have been essential for the survival of your forebears, your own survival depends on being able to keep it under control. And the simplest way to do so is with drugs.

The best-known drugs that dampen sympathetic arousal are the so-called *beta-receptor blockers*. To exert any effect, the catecholamines have to switch on particular reactions in the tissue cells of, say, the heart or blood vessels. To do so they first have to fit into particular gaps or 'receptors' on the cell surface, much as a key fits into a lock. There are two types and those on the surface of the heart are known as the *beta-receptors*, to distinguish them from the other, alpha group. Drugs which block beta-receptors will keep most of the catecholamines out of the 'keyhole'. They are therefore known, appropriately enough, as beta-receptor blockers, or *beta-blockers* for short. They are a very important type of medication, used to control arrhythmias, angina and hypertension. And they certainly reduce the catecholamine response.

For example, we know that racing drivers show a dramatic catecholamine increase during a competition. Didier Pironi at Monaco in 1981 had a pulse rate between 190 and 210 for the whole race of nearly two hours. Such a dangerously high rate can be brought down by blocking the beta-receptors. For obvious reasons there haven't been any attempts to study drug effects under Grand Prix conditions. But racing drivers have been followed over practice laps, both with and without medication. Beta-blockade brought their heart rates down by nearly a half, back to near-normal levels. And free fatty acids, which also increased steeply during a fast drive, showed no rise at all when the drivers were given their beta-blocking drugs.

We also know what happens to young doctors when they have to describe their work to their senior colleagues. Some of the doctors followed in one study had heart rates up to 180 per minute, with marked rhythm disturbances and rises in both free fatty acids and triglycerides when they came to present their results. A single dose of a beta-blocker taken before their next speaking assignment largely prevented any increase in heart rate, as well as greatly reducing the arrhythmias and fat breakdown.

The same thing happens with smokers. Carruthers found that both low and high nicotine cigarettes produced a rise in heart rate, blood pressure and free fatty acids. But a single beta-blocker dose taken in advance stopped them all from rising above normal levels.

If beta-blockers are so good at reducing the effects of catecholamine stimulation, are they perhaps the answer to the overdriver's problem? Should the chronic Type A1, who seems to live for the noradrenaline highs, simply take a pill a day so that he can go on enjoying the stimulation but avoid the consequences?

We will look at this possibility as part of the all-important question of treatment. Some specialists are certainly considering such an approach. But others are more cautious. Beta-blockers only block the receptors. They don't block the catecholamines. Adrenaline and noradrenaline are still released in the same (perhaps even larger) quantities, in response to the same emotional or physical challenge. But does it matter, if they've been 'uncoupled' from most of the effects they usually produce? The answer is that it might.

Then again, we've only looked at the sympathetic side. But there's another aspect to the overdriver's problem resulting from the action of the vagus, and beta-blockade has no effect on that at all.

You will remember that the parasympathetic is the heart's braking system. And we seem to go around with the brake on for most of the time. The speed the heart would beat if there were no nerves controlling it is actually faster than the heart rate most of us have at rest. So the vagus is normally in command. And if the vagal influence becomes stronger than normal, the slowing of the heart can be very marked indeed. This probably explains the fainting attacks that some of us experience if we're suddenly exposed to unpleasant situations. The way that some medical students pass out in the operating theatre is a joke to their seniors: 'You'll never be a surgeon if you faint at the sight of blood.' And young police officers sometimes keel over when they attend their first post-mortem.

Occasionally, the heart may slow down so much that it stops altogether. Dr Gottfried Härtel, a cardiologist at the University of Helsinki, tells the story of two Finnish sisters, who received a visit from one sister's fiancé. He had bad news for her, so bad that she suddenly went pale, stopped breathing and fell over. The other sister, who had seen what happened, also collapsed. They were rushed to hospital, where they both died, one from fibrillation, the other because her heart had simply stopped. Both were only twenty-two years old.

Deaths like these are rare, because the human heart takes some stopping. Even so, the power of the vagus to slow down the heart is impressive, even in surroundings that would normally send it racing. For example, imagine a visit to the dentist. The anxiety that you feel sitting in the outer office and walking towards the chair is quite enough to raise your adrenaline and your pulse rate. But close study of a group of nurses having dental treatment in London showed that as they got into the chair, their heart rates actually fell. Their pulses stayed low during the local anaesthetic and the drilling and only rose again once they knew it was finished. By contrast, their blood adrenaline levels were raised the whole time and reached a peak during the treatment. The uncontrollable, unpleasant event simply caused the vagus to override the sympathetic system.

The same research group described a parachutist whose heart rate and adrenaline levels were being monitored as he made his jump. During his descent his pulse was up to 185. Unfortunately, on landing he broke his ankle. Within a few seconds the rate fell to 60, although his plasma adrenaline was still well above normal. Again, in response to the unpleasant event, his parasympathetic system simply took over.

You don't even have to live through the event to activate the vagus. Simply watching it is enough. Some of the research team who did the dental study were interested to know what effect violent films had on your cardiovascular system. They knew, for example, that people sometimes fainted during especially unpleasant scenes. To find out, they took groups of volunteers to see *Soldier Blue* and *A Clockwork Orange*, two of the most violent films around in the early 1970s when the study was done. Measuring heart rates and collecting blood and urine samples in a cinema isn't easy, but with great ingenuity they pre-booked a block of seats and wired themselves up to a central recording box before the feature started. The wires were covered by sweaters or jackets. Samples were obtained only five minutes after the end of *Soldier Blue*, thanks to a cooperative cinema manager who allowed them to use his office.

The results were striking. Adrenaline levels in urine were almost twice as high after the film as they had been before. Noradrenaline levels were also raised. Free fatty acids were doubled as well. Despite this, heart rates measured during the most violent sequences were actually lower than when the volunteers had been resting before the performance. And these changes occurred even though most of the volunteers were involved in some branch of medicine, and were no strangers to death and maiming.

So although your sympathetic system is switched on when you have to make some active response to a threat or challenge, it's your parasympathetic that takes over when you are faced with a situation that you can't do anything about.

The brain region that takes command when conditions become uncertain stops the action that you are currently engaged in – which isn't having any impact on the problem – and says: 'Slow everything down for a while, look around, and see if there's a better way you could be dealing with this.' If there isn't, the brain says: 'Maybe you won't be able to handle it at the moment. But keep your eyes open. Perhaps the situation will change.' This reaction, the complete opposite of fight-or-flight, is generally known as *conservation-withdrawal*.

It is a sensible way to respond. You could destroy yourself by grappling time and again with the same unyielding problem, be it job loss, illness or bereavement. But there's no guarantee that you'll like it. Male apes or even male mice, put in a withdrawn state because a more aggressive male has taken over the colony, seem demoralized and may even die. Human beings who are similarly withdrawn can't help being depressed either, and the depression brings its own problems.

While active coping involves the release of noradrenaline

from nerve endings and adrenaline from the adrenals, conservation-withdrawal has its own adrenal hormone – indeed more than one. The one we'll concentrate on is called *cortisol*. It is normally secreted in periodic squirts, and more is shot into the blood stream in the morning than during the rest of the day. But when conditions are uncertain, cortisol is released at an increased rate. It goes up when we are faced with new situations, and it goes up and stays up when we can't find an appropriate way to respond. It is released by other triggers as well, but that would take us too far from our story.

Cortisol has many effects. One of its functions is to prevent allergy and inflammation. But it also stimulates the breakdown of fats, raising the risk of atheroma. It increases the number of platelets and also their stickiness, so it boosts the chance of blood clotting. And when the sympathetic system is activated at the same time, it makes blood vessels contract more readily. So any increase in cortisol may be as bad a coronary risk as an increase in catecholamines. And it is a worse risk for other diseases.

If cortisol is the main hormone for withdrawal, and the withdrawn person feels distressed, then you might expect cortisol to be an indicator of distress. And you'd be right.

I mentioned Marianne Frankenhaeuser's study where volunteers had to do a monotonous job but at the same time they had to keep alert, like someone who spends his time watching a set of dials. If the dial-watcher's attention starts to wander, the result can be Three Mile Island. They also had to react to conflicting inputs when the names of colours were flashed on a screen, but the lettering was in a different colour from the word that it spelled. The problem was to ignore the word and shout out the colour, and they had to do it quickly. They were asked how they felt after each test. At the same time urine samples were collected to see how their hormones were responding.

The vigilance task produced both effort and distress. The volunteers said that they were tense and had to concentrate while they were doing it, but at the same time it made them bored, impatient, tired and irritable. In these conditions both adrenaline and cortisol went up. They also did a button-pressing task that depended on the speed of their reactions. But they were allowed to do that at their own pace. If they felt it was getting away from them they could stop, and start again at a slower rate. They still had to concentrate but this time they felt none of the distress that they had before. During this task their adrenaline levels also rose, but their cortisol values actually fell to lower levels than before they started.

So a task over which they had little control put their cortisols up, but one that they could control well, and which gave them a feeling of mastery, actually reduced it. The catecholamine and cortisol reactions had different triggers.

Frankenhaeuser's group looked at this reaction-time test more closely. It involved sitting in front of two rows of coloured buttons. When a button in one row lit up the volunteer had to find and press a button of the same colour in the other row as quickly as possible. They were allowed to practise before the start, and every five minutes they could change the speed at which the buttons lit up if they wanted to. After a while, they had almost complete control.

The question was whether Type As would select a higher speed than Type Bs, and if so would they make more mistakes? So the test was repeated using twenty-four Type As and a similar number of Bs (as defined by a Swedish version of the JAS). As you might guess, the As did choose to work faster than the Bs and in this test they consistently scored higher than the Bs as well. Both groups said that they experienced effort (the men more so than the women) but little distress. And their urinary values bore this out. Adrenaline increased (again, more for the men than the women) but at the same time cortisol actually fell. The researchers summed it up: 'The heightened catecholamine level reflects the challenge to perform well, while the lower cortisol level reflects the experience of being in control of the situation.'

These findings fit with other measurements taken under more searching conditions. Cortisol levels in some NASA astronauts (men with the 'right stuff') were said to be so low that mission control wondered whether the machine was measuring them properly. It seems that they were finding the mission so exhilarating that they felt no distress at all. Similar findings were reported among helicopter pilots in Vietnam. Men flying medical sorties had a poor chance of coming back. So you would expect their adrenals to be working overtime. But the group who were looked at had particularly high self-esteem. They knew their job was vital. They were bringing back wounded men who would otherwise certainly have died. The sense of achievement that this gave them was apparently enough to suppress their adrenal distress, and cortisol-like secretions remained low.

But what happens in real-life situations when we feel effort and distress together, or one straight after the other? It can happen many times a day, and it can be, quite literally, bad news.

Dr George Engel of the University of Rochester in New York has been interested for many years in what happens when the sympathetic or parasympathetic systems are over-activated. The most dramatic result is sudden death, and he has collected a large number of newspaper reports of such deaths following some event that was impossible for the victim to ignore. Usually they involved either overwhelming excitement or total giving up.

For example, he quotes the case of the army captain who commanded the ceremonial troop at the funeral of President Kennedy. Although he was only twenty-seven this officer died ten days after the President, apparently as the result of an arrhythmia. A forty-year-old man died in the street as he knelt beside his son whose motorbike had crashed. A middle-aged physician learned that he was not going to get the job left vacant by his retiring chief. After a meeting with the chief, he became so angry that he fell down dead, the victim of ventricular fibrillation. People have died watching horror scenes on television but others have collapsed after getting good news. One seventy-five-year-old man died after winning $1500 for a $2 bet.

While all these cases involve *either* action or withdrawal, Engel's researches have also revealed a group of people who experienced both at the same time. One middle-aged man died when his mother refused to pay his gambling debts, as she had always done in the past. But this time the mob was after him. With his last escape route blocked he slumped dead at his desk, the victim of an infarction. Another man of similar age found life unbearable in the town he was living in. He arranged to move, but just before he left, a major difficulty also developed in the town he was planning to move to. Not knowing what to do, he got on the train. Unable to resolve the problem on the journey, he got out at a station stop half-way to his destination. When the conductor called 'All aboard' his desperation reached its peak. He dropped dead on the platform – infarction again.

Both of these men were threatened by an uncertainty that couldn't be resolved: for one where to get the money that would save him; for the other, whether to go or to stay. In these circumstances, Engel suggests, the sympathetic and parasympathetic systems, which usually act in opposition (remember the accelerator and the brake?), actually get turned on at the same time. It is like hitting both pedals together. The fight-or-flight reaction is triggered while the victim is paralysed by uncertainty. His circulation, which normally shunts blood to where it is most needed, simply fails. At best he faints, because the brain's blood supply suffers a temporary fall. At worst he may die, because the heart itself is starved of oxygen.

And sometimes we have only ourselves to blame if escape is impossible. Many men feel a need to exaggerate their bravery, and disprove any hint of weakness. As a result, they volunteer to be first into some unfamiliar, frightening or painful situation. Their response to medical treatment is an example. That's why hospital faints – when the needle hits the vein – are more frequent in men than women.

You can't place too much reliance on newspaper reports – Engel admits as much. But the events leading up to bouts of fibrillation have also been looked at in much greater detail, and the results are similar. For example, 100 patients at Harvard who had heart attacks bad enough to put them in hospital, but not bad enough to kill them, were interviewed in depth about what had happened during the previous twenty-four hours. More than one in five admitted to some major psychological disturbance – perhaps a bereavement, a business failure or a bout of anger, excitement, fear or depression. One man's heart had started racing during an argument with his wife. Another's took off when his wife left his hospital bedside. When asked what was the matter, he said he was afraid that she would be attacked on the street.

Questioning patients in St Paul, Minnesota, who had congestive heart failure, in which the heart can't handle its fluid load properly, also showed that nearly half of them had experienced some emotional disturbance that made them bad enough to be hospitalized. With one middle-aged man it was a change of landlord in his apartment block. He had got on well with the old one, but the new one was hostile and unhelpful. Another, older patient, had seen all the houses in his block knocked down, one by one. But what had put him in the hospital wasn't the sight of his own home going under the bulldozer, but the immense and unexpected relief he had felt on hearing that it was being allowed to remain standing.

Sudden death at work can also be caused by psychological triggers. A research group in Manitoba followed the lives of nearly a thousand World War II pilots over thirty years to see what they died of. Some one hundred and fifty of them were victims of sudden coronary death and more than a quarter of them died on Mondays – far more than you'd expect by chance. There seems little doubt that the hassle involved in coming back to the office or the factory after the comparative calm of the weekend may trigger a clutch of arrhythmias.

There's just one last observation that I have to make about the withdrawal reaction, which is at present largely speculation but is too important to ignore. It is that while overdriving your sympathetic system will damage your heart, years of withdrawal may reduce your defence against cancer.

Large quantities of cortisol are released from your adrenal cortex during periods of depression and helplessness. Cortisol has an anti-inflammatory action; it reduces the number of white blood cells. But some of these cells are involved in defending your body against attack. They make up one of the arms of your immune system, and any reduction could leave you vulnerable to foreign cells. Worse perhaps, since your immune system is also constantly on the look-out for any of the body's own cells that are becoming malignant, reducing its effectiveness by prolonged releases of cortisol may lower our cancer defences too.

This is exactly what happens in experimental animals. If mice are made helpless by constantly rotating them on a gramophone turntable, their cortisol levels rise. As a result, the number of white cells and their production rate both fall. If tumours are transplanted into mice that have been treated in this way, they are more likely to grow than they would in normal animals.

And what about people? White cells have been reported

to fall following overwork and are less active after bereavements. Obviously, we can't relate this directly to the growth of tumours, and the evidence in man has to be indirect. Even so, it is very suggestive.

In a long-term study of graduates from Johns Hopkins Medical School in Baltimore, the cause of death in alumni in their thirties and forties was compared with questionnaires that they had filled in as young men, questionnaires that gave information particularly about their levels of tension. The results still need further checking, but it seems that individuals destined to suffer from cancer admitted, all those years before, that they often felt exhaustion and fatigue, and that they checked and rechecked their work to make sure that it was right.

Even more interesting were their personal relationships. Those who went on to develop cancer felt themselves less close to their parents, particularly their fathers, than their more healthy contemporaries. It may be that as children they tried to make closer contact but were continually rebuffed, until they eventually gave up and retreated into themselves.

Speculation? Perhaps, but the results of a detailed survey of over a thousand people in a small town in Yugoslavia certainly make it all seem possible. In 1965 they too answered a questionnaire designed to see whether they were submissive, non-aggressive citizens, who deferred to those more dominant than themselves, or whether, on the contrary, they were active competitive drivers, anxious to maintain control over situations and more likely to repress other people than to be repressed by them.

They were followed up until 1976, during which time the appearance of any cancer or other disease was recorded. And guess what? There was a link between the appearance of cancer and the way that they projected themselves. Cancers were more frequent among those who were described as 'receivers of repression' than among the 'emitters of repression' who presumably ordered them around. The emitters, by contrast, seemed to have higher levels of circulatory and other diseases.

So those of us in 'no exit' situations, like bereavement, or the loss of a job at a particularly bad time, might be at higher risk because of the resulting feelings of isolation, helplessness and despair that they bring. And those who consistently suppress their own feelings and defer to others may be in the same boat.

We may therefore have to live with the cynics, who tell us that the world is perfectly balanced. On the one hand are the aggressive and repressing, who exert their will on everyone else and get coronaries as a result. On the other are the passive and repressed, who sit there and take it all and end up with cancer. All you have to decide is which you'd rather be.

However, they forget the majority of us who lie somewhere in between. Even worse, they ignore the possibility that both the repressers and the repressed may be able to pull themselves round to normality. Or rather, to sanity. Because normality, for the overdriver at least, is a series of highs and lows that no one could describe as sane.

5. Superpong and Hot Responders

We now know enough about the nervous system to ask why Type A is a risk factor for coronary disease. What is it about the Type A's behaviour or his beliefs that eventually stops his heart and why are some more at risk than others?

Firstly, Type As get as tired as anyone else. But to get the job done they deny their fatigue and carry on driving themselves, with promises like: 'I'll take some time off when I've just finished this.' They also deny that there is anything wrong with them when they have what they believe to be minor aches and pains. Even a pain in the chest may be ignored – remember George and Irving? So Type As may be coronary prone because they drive themselves to exhaustion and ignore warning signs that would make the Type B slow down or visit his doctor.

But there are other, more distinct links between Type A and heart disease. Many large hospitals can now measure the extent to which your coronary arteries may be blocked by atheroma. The procedure, which is not particularly pleasant, and not without its risks, is known as coronary angiography. A tube is guided under X-ray through your major arteries until it lies close to the coronaries. X-ray fluid is then delivered from it into the coronary arteries themselves. Films are taken, which tell those who are trained to read them by how much each coronary artery is blocked, and where the blockage is located.

On several occasions, before angiography, patients have had their Type A status measured, and more arterial narrowing was found among the As than the Bs. In one particular investigation in 1978, patients with more than 75 per cent narrowing of at least one coronary artery also had high scores on a pyschological test of hostility that had nothing to do with being Type A. When they were also given the structured interview, the hostility component of that came out high as well. Finding such high scores among Type As with major coronary disease raised the possibility that their advanced atherosclerosis might somehow result from their hostility level.

But before we conclude that the subject is all sewn up – Type A producing atheroma and atheroma leading to death – I have to say that other cardiologists in leading medical centres have found no link at all between Type A and coronary atheroma. Angiography showed coronary patients to have narrowed arteries, but the narrowing bore no relation to their Type A status. The mystery gets greater when we learn that two such studies, one positive and one negative, were conducted within a few miles of each other in two hospitals in Boston. When the research teams compared notes, neither could fault the other's methods or conclusions. But they couldn't find any way of reconciling their results either.

One question that is often asked is why we spend all our time concentrating on coronary disease. Type A is a common enough behaviour and you might expect it to be related to other diseases too. But so far it doesn't seem to be. The only other disease that shows an increase among Type As appears to be stroke. Some doctors don't believe that the story will end there. Take gastric ulcer patients, for example. Many of them show a time-urgent, hostile approach to life, and it is possible that the Type A pattern might be responsible for at least some of their gastric problems. We shall see. Otherwise there seems to be only one extra hazard that we have to take notice of, and it will surprise no one. Type As with high JAS scores on Speed and Impatience have an increased risk of death from accidents or violence.

But what is the basic link between Type A and the nervous system? The answer to that can't be found from the JAS. It comes from looking closely at the structured interview. When Dr Karen Matthews and Professor David Glass were at the University of Texas in Austin, they worked with Ray Rosenman to break down the structured interview (much as David Jenkins had broken down the JAS). They found five components: competitive drive, impatience, past achievement, non-job achievement and speed. Then they looked at how these features were shared among the heart disease victims in the Western Collaborative Study. Only the first two, competitive drive and impatience, were linked with coronary disease. If you don't suffer from either of them, then tackling problems faster than most other people, or taking pride in a string of past achievements, apparently makes you no more liable to heart disease than the next man.

And it was David Glass, after he had moved from Texas to New York, who was among the first to show what a combination of competition and impatience can do to your sympathetic system. Glass had been involved in Type A research from an early stage. Like Friedman and Rosenman, he reasoned that the Type A would show his true self when he was faced with some challenge to his self-esteem. One of Glass's main interests was how such behaviour influenced the release of adrenaline and noradrenaline, a subject about which there was very little information.

Back in the 1960s, the San Francisco group had looked at noradrenaline excretion in the urine and found no difference between Type As and Bs in the quantity they produced overnight. However, in urine collected after working hours, Type As had more nonadrenaline than Bs. At the time, this fitted very well with the idea of aggressive, time-urgent behaviour producing the so-called aggressive catecholamine.

By the mid-1970s, Rosenman and Friedman had gone further. They had decided to see what effect competition had on catecholamine levels. Fifteen pairs of middle-aged Type A volunteers were made to compete with each other, trying to solve a series of puzzles to win a bottle of wine. Blood samples were taken before, during and after the fifteen-minute contest. While there were no differences between As and Bs before the competition, the increase in noradrenaline during the test was higher among the As. Again, this seemed good evidence of sympathetic over-arousal.

Unfortunately, though both of these experiments were very suggestive and very important, neither of them answered the question completely, because of problems with the way they were set up. When the urine studies were done it was difficult even to measure small amounts of catecholamines accurately. And the competitions involved repeated blood sampling with a hypodermic needle, something that might itself make a sensitive person's catecholamines shoot up. They needed repeating and extending. Glass himself has never claimed that his own experiments are free from mistakes, but they gave a fuller, more clear and convincing picture of the Type A's biochemical reactions to the problems of everyday life.

In his best-known work, published in 1980 when he was at the City University of New York, Glass managed to gain the cooperation of a group of middle-aged Transit Authority workers – motormen, conductors and repair men – to act as subjects for his experiments. He wanted to put them into a competitive situation, in which they would strive to achieve something and at the same time feel hassled and irritated. To do this in a laboratory, even one on 42nd Street in New York, is more difficult than you could ever imagine. After a short time, most volunteers get quite used to the lab surroundings and the tasks they are being given to do. Their reactions start to get blunt, unlike the real-life situation on the street outside, where a constant stream of new challenges means that they have to stay sharp the whole time.

One task that he thought would keep them competing and involved was a TV game – Superpong – a form of televised hockey, where you use a control lever to put the electronic ball through your opponent's goal. And to produce the irritation, what better than a harassing opponent, a big-mouth who not only plays the game well, but never lets you forget it?

The volunteers turned up at a laboratory and went through the usual structured interview to decide who was Type A and Type B. Later, they had a tube placed in an arm vein so that blood could be withdrawn at any time, without the need for repeated punctures. They were fitted with a blood pressure cuff and a device for measuring their heart rate, and after ten minutes of rest listening to Mantovani they were set to compete at Superpong against an opponent, the prize being a $25 gift certificate to Macy's Department Store.

What they didn't know was that the opponent had spent a whole summer training at the game. He could win (or lose) any one of the nine game series at will, and he always ended up taking the certificate. With half the Transit workers he deliberately set out to hassle them with remarks like: 'Can't you keep your eye on the ball?' 'Maybe I'd better give you a few points' and 'Christ, you're not even trying'. I have often wondered how he got to the end of the series with a full set of teeth. With the other subjects he played in silence. And the effects of his interaction were dramatic.

Both Type A and Type B volunteers got sufficiently involved in the game for their heart rate and blood pressure to rise. The increases were similar for both groups. It wasn't possible to tell the As from the Bs as long as the opponent kept his mouth shut. But, as soon as he started to hassle, the As showed greater rises in pumping (systolic) blood pressure, heart rate and adrenaline levels (with smaller rises in noradrenaline) than when they were playing in silence. The extra dimension provided by the opponent's commentary was just what it took to get a maximum response.

Glass has suggested that the Type A may spend much of his ordinary life in his 'hyper-responsive' state and we know very well the effects that such sympathetic arousal can have on your cardiovascular system. Plaques, arrhythmias and blood clots are just three of the probable results of winding up for fight-or-flight, and then finding nothing to release it on.

But what happens when, despite his striving, the Type A's efforts simply don't work – the problem is too difficult, or it simply can't be solved that way? Then he's likely to become dejected and depressed, a pattern that looks very like conservation-withdrawal. He becomes, in Glass's phrase, 'hypo-responsive'. At that point cortisol may become the important hormone, with its effects on atherosclerosis and the immune system. Such swings between one system and the other and the chance of both of them being switched on at once, have an all-too-familiar ring.

We know that the Type A1 needs very little to set him off, and this experiment by David Glass shows just what can do it best. Competition with a dash of contempt is something that many of us are exposed to every day, and it puts the Type A's sympathetic system on full throttle. But what is it in his make-up that makes him react in this way?

The answer to that was found by Dr Theodore M. Dembroski of Eckert College in St Petersburg, Florida. It fits well with the atheroma story and with Friedman's core beliefs. More than anything else, what trips the Type A's switch is his hostility.

Dembroski took university student volunteers and classified them Type A or B by the interview. He then gave them two tasks. The first was to hold their right hand for seventy-five seconds in a bucket of iced water. This 'cold pressor' test has been used for years to activate the sympathetic system and it does it very well. A minute with your hand in the ice bucket seems like a very long time – try it yourself. Their other task was less painful. It involved them reacting to green and red flashing lights as quickly as possible.

But more important than the tasks themselves were the conditions in which they were done. The students were told either that they were common enough tests, which anyone could do without much effort, or else that they were real challenges, needing considerable will-power to bear the iced water and quick responses to keep ahead of the flashing lights. During each trial the experimenter measured their heart rate and blood pressure responses.

The Type As tended to have bigger reactions to both tasks than Type Bs. And telling the volunteers that the task was difficult also generally produced a greater response than telling them it was easy. So all in all, Type As showed more reaction than Bs, and highly challenged As showed the greatest reactions of all. Predictable you might think – but the most interesting feature couldn't have been predicted.

Dembroski's group have made a fine-grained analysis of the structured interview, both the voice style when the subject replies (its loudness, speed and acceleration) and the content of what he actually says. It was they who produced the 1–5 scoring system that many others now use. As a result they were able to identify one particular feature, a mixture of competitiveness, hostility, speed and impatience, that they called *hostility/competition*. The students were divided on the basis of whether they were low or high on this characteristic, and the division revealed a crucial difference in their reactions.

When they thought the tasks were easy, Type As who were low on hostility reacted much like Type Bs. Only when they

were told it was important did they react more than the Type
B volunteers. But highly hostile As showed a maximum
response whether they had been told the task was important
or not. They had only one reaction for all conditions – 'go
for it'.

If we apply these research findings to real life, Dembroski
suggested that the world should be divided not into two
groups but into three. First are the Type Bs, who need a very
high level of challenge to arouse them to the point where they
might do themselves any damage. Then come the low-hostile
As, who react more easily. But most reactive of all are the
high-hostile As who are quite unselective in what turns them
on. Even a trivial task is a major challenge *to them*. They react
the same way, whatever the provocation, and give
themselves the highest coronary risk. Problems that many of
us are able to take in our stride (the need to change your plans
from one day to the next, or sometimes to accept frustration
and disappointment) are problems that have a major impact
on high-hostile As. So it's perhaps not surprising that
hostility has links with disease that are quite independent of
any Type A pattern.

For example, research workers in Detroit recently looked
at how anger interacts with three other important causes of
high blood pressure or hypertension. The three are sex, race
and the type of environment in which you live. We know that
men have more hypertensive disease than women, and blacks
in many parts of the United States have higher blood
pressures than whites. People who live in socially deprived
neighbourhoods also tend to have higher pressures, probably
because having to react to challenges every day keeps it at a
higher level than it otherwise would be.

The Detroit survey team measured people's blood
pressures at home. And at the same time they asked them a
series of questions about how they would normally respond
to being challenged or attacked by, say, their boss, a

policeman or even by their spouse or children. Would they get mad and show it (getting their 'anger out'), or would they keep it to themselves (keeping their 'anger in')? When the results were analysed, they showed that 'anger in' was itself a risk factor for hypertension. It produced about the same risk as sex, race or neighbourhood. Each one increased the chance of being hypertensive, and for black men in poor neighbourhoods the risk was increased nearly sixfold.

Now you can't do anything about your sex or race, and you may not be able to do much about where you live. From these findings it seems that getting your anger out, instead of bottling it up, may protect your arteries. But it's far better to try to see the world in a way that doesn't get you angry at all. A tall order you may think. And it is, as we'll see when we look later at ways of trying to do it. But more and more studies like this are telling us that we have to try.

One of David Glass's own research projects looked at individuals whose blood pressure shoots up when they have to perform a difficult task like subtracting numbers in their head, or dealing with conflicting information. These 'high responders' also felt more anger, irritation and tension after the conflict was over, than did a group of 'low responders' whose blood pressure had shown little change.

But there's more to hostility than meets the eye. Whether you get angry may depend on the situation. But it also depends on your previous experience. Glass didn't find that his more hostile and competitive Type A subjects (as judged by the structured interview) necessarily had the greatest responses. So they differed from Dembroski's group of high-hostile Type As, whose blood pressure went up even when the challenge was minimal. But Dembroski had used college students aged between eighteen and twenty-six. Glass's subjects were New York police and firemen in their early forties, men who prided themselves on keeping their cool and having their feelings well under control. In this they may have been like the 'anger in' group in Detroit, keeping their irritation well hidden and not allowing themselves any outward display of hostility.

In any case, as Glass has pointed out, we need a much clearer distinction between anger, hostility and aggression. We use the three words as though they meant the same thing. But they don't. All of them are generally directed outwards, towards other people. But they can be directed inwards too. And to fire them in either direction is a luxury that we really can't afford.

If you doubt it you have only to look at two pieces of research from North Carolina. We have glanced briefly at one of them already – hostility and atheroma. Dr Redford B. Williams and his colleagues examined over four hundred heart patients who attended the Duke University Medical Center in 1976–7 for angiography to see whether their coronary arteries were blocked. Every patient in the series had a structured interview to assess his or her Type A status, and their feelings of hostility were recorded on a separate questionnaire.

This particular set of questions is well known to psychologists. It has been around since the 1950s, and forms part of the hugely comprehensive Minnesota Multiphasic Personality Inventory, or MMPI. Participants are asked whether they agree or disagree with statements like: 'Some of my family have habits that bother and annoy me very much', 'I have at times had to be rough with people who were rude or annoying' or 'I have often met people supposed to be experts who were no better than I'.

The results of the SI and the hostility scale were then compared with the angiographic findings. As we've seen, to make the comparison easier, the research team concentrated on patients who had at least one artery blocked by 75 per cent somewhere along its length. More of them were found to be Type A than Type B. But more of them had high scores on the MMPI hostility questionnaire as well. Indeed, when the computer analyses were completed, it was found that Type A and hostility both predicted coronary blockage, and hostility actually predicted it better. The results were true both for men and women and, of course, the risk factors interacted. So the chance of a non-hostile, non-Type A woman having a severely blocked artery was only 13 per cent, while for a hostile Type A man it rose to 82 per cent.

These findings obviously provide important guidelines about who will benefit from angiography. The chances of finding a blockage in a low-hostile Type B might be so remote that both doctor and patient should question whether the procedure is worth the risks and the expense involved. They also point to the same conclusion as the Detroit results. Some of the current effort and considerable funding that are presently going into coronary prevention should be focused on altering patients' anger and hostility levels.

The same message shouts even louder from a second piece of research by Williams and his colleagues. You will remember that what Friedman and Rosenman needed to convince the medical profession of the dangers of Type A was a so-called 'prospective study' to measure the risk factor in a group of people, follow them over the years and see what happened to them. The North Carolina group had the same view about hostility, but setting up a study like the WCGS was a non-starter. Fortunately, the basis for a prospective study had been laid many years before, almost by accident. Between 1954 and 1959, medical students at the University had filled in bits of the MMPI as part of their normal training. Their answers were still on file. If it were possible to locate those who were living, to determine the cause of death of the others, and to relate the findings to their MMPI replies of twenty years before, then it might be possible to assess the long-term effects of hostility on well-being.

Accordingly, in 1981 a health questionnaire was sent to all

the University of North Carolina medical school alumni who had taken the MMPI. Replies came back from over two hundred and fifty. With their permission their health records, particularly for cardiovascular disease, were matched against their hostility levels, rated either *high* or *low*. Coronary heart disease was nearly five times more frequent in the high-hostile responders. Closer analysis showed that the effect was genuine, and not due to differences in their age or smoking habits. When the research team examined the records of those who had died in the interim, they found that high hostility scores predicted mortality not only from coronary disease, but from other causes, including cancer and accidents as well, so that total deaths were six times more frequent among the high scorers.

This effect of hostility on non-coronary deaths can best be understood by looking at the attitudes of those doctors with high scores. They distrusted everyone. They thought that other people were selfish and inconsiderate, that they would exploit you if they could, and that they deserved to be punished. It's an attitude that reminds us very much of the Type A1's view of the rest of the world. But it's arrived at here using one of the best known of psychological tests – a test that was published before Type A ever saw the light. The way in which the SI and the MMPI, two tests with little in common, reveal the *same* core beliefs (and the dangers they produce) is really most impressive.

With attitudes like these, the high scorer will obviously distance himself from other people. More important perhaps, they will distance themselves from him. The result is that as well as disturbing his physiology, he is depriving himself of the human contact that all of us need, not only for our comfort, but for our continued survival. The high-hostile individual simply kicks away one of his life supports.

The type of hostility thrown up by the MMPI overlaps with the structured interview, but it's not quite the same. As well as distrust, Type As show active aggression. But they're not the only ones who show over-reactive heart rate or blood pressure or adrenaline responses. Overdrivers who aren't Type A (at least not obviously so) respond the same way if the challenge is right.

David Glass found this in his anger study. His main interest was to see whether men with exaggerated reactions to one type of test responded the same way to another. He already knew that some Type As didn't show the responses to challenge that you would expect, whereas some Type Bs did. It seems that heredity or maybe your early environment may dispose you to be an over-reactor (what I've called an overdriver), whatever your Type A status.

Glass had his New York Police and Fire Department volunteers go through a mental arithmetic test. They had to subtract 13 from 1179, then from the figure that was left, and so on. They had to shout out their answers every two seconds, in time with a ticking metronome, and occasionally an investigator in the next room would come on the intercom and tell them that they were falling behind. Throughout the test their heart rate and blood pressure were being recorded.

Not surprisingly, this test was enough to raise nearly all their pumping blood pressures (again, try it for yourself, even without the metronome). Those who responded with sharp rises were described as 'high reactors' in contrast to the 'low reactors' who showed lesser response. All of them then went through a Type A structured interview.

Some months later they came back to try a second test – one that we've seen before. The name of a colour appeared on a screen. It was printed in a coloured ink, but the word and the ink colour weren't the same. Glass's volunteers had to ignore the word and shout out the colour it was printed in. But the words only stayed on the screen for about half a second. And to make things more difficult, they had to wear headphones. On the sound track they also heard the names of colours, synchronized in time with those flashing in front of them. But the sound track was also out of phase, so that the printed word, the ink colour and the spoken word were never the same.

As if the problem weren't complicated enough, two minutes into the ten-minute trial the researcher on the intercom told them that they would have to start again – they were going too slowly. During this whole harrowing incident, blood pressures and heart rate were recorded, and a blood sample taken at the end was compared with one taken before the start, to look for any change in catecholamines.

When the arithmetic test was compared with the colour-slide results, Glass found that high reactors on the first test also showed increased heart rate and blood pressure during the second. They had raised levels of noradrenaline as well, when compared to the low reactors. So the pattern was stable. High reactors were still high reactors when they were measured some months later, and involved in a different task. But their Type A scores had little effect. High reactors were no more likely to be Type A than B.

This shouldn't come as much of a surprise. The high reactors were originally selected because of their response to arithmetic, not because of anything to do with their Type A. And both As and Bs may have been stretched so far by the arithmetic test that any differences simply disappeared. Even Type Bs can be switched on if they are provoked far enough. The difference is one of degree, not of kind.

Indeed, some of Glass's own research has shown that in the right conditions, Bs may react even more than As.

Many of those who have worked with Type A patients have noticed that because they pride themselves on having all situations under control and on being able to handle any crisis, they feel that they have to show a brave face to the world and suppress any outward feelings of anger, fear or distress. Accordingly, Glass's colleague, Dr William F.

Hilton, thought that Type As might be less reactive than Bs when it comes to expressing emotion.

He asked a group of A and B subjects to spend three minutes remembering situations that in the past had made them angry, afraid or distressed. At the end of the three minutes reliving each emotion for themselves, they were asked to describe the situation as though they were talking to a sympathetic friend, so that the friend could really feel what it had been like. After each period, a blood sample was taken and compared with one drawn before the session began, to look for catecholamine changes.

The results confirmed the prediction. Type Bs showed greater rises in noradrenaline than As both when reliving and when retelling the emotional incidents. To confirm that Type As lower responses really did result from their suppressing their emotions, Hilton had video tapes made of the volunteers as they thought about and described each incident. The As' facial expressions changed much less than the Bs'. If we believe that what shows on your face is any guide to what's going on inside, then the Type As, who were showing fewer signs of emotion, were presumably feeling less of it as well.

But periods of emotion are not the only times that Type Bs may be more reactive. Dr Margaret A. Chesney and her colleagues at SRI International, a leading research institute in Stanford, California, looked at the working environment of nearly four hundred white-collar men at the Lockheed Missile and Space Company. More particularly, they examined the workers' reactions to their environment, as measured by their blood pressure, heart rate and a variety of biochemical studies. With Ray Rosenman, then a senior research physician at SRI, they did structured interviews for Type A as well.

They found that those Type As who thought their occupational settings encouraged them to make their own decisions, to take initiatives and to carry responsibility, had lower blood pressures than those who didn't. Nothing surprising there – it fits well with the notion of Type A as dominant and self-confident. But Type Bs had *higher* blood pressures in jobs that called for independent action. For them, pressures were lower in situations that encouraged dependence on others. It seemed that they might actually be at higher risk of developing heart disease in settings where they were expected to take the lead. And attempts to restructure the work environment so as to lessen the risk of CHD would have to take these differences into account.

So we can see overdrive continuing to separate from Type A. Some Type As may not be over-reactors (though many of them are). And some of those with an over-reactive sympathetic system may not be Type As either, or at least, they may have it so well hidden that even an experienced interviewer can't detect it. Those who are both have a real problem. Their Type A behaviour takes them constantly into situations that activate their nervous responses. At least that's the best explanation of the dangers of the Type A pattern that we have at present – and I believe that more research will confirm it.

But some experts believe that we shouldn't place too much emphasis on Type A. What we should go for is the response pattern itself. For example, Professor Robert S. Eliot, until recently Director of the Cardiovascular Center at the University of Nebraska at Omaha, examined a group of senior executives of the Western Electric Company. He followed their cardiovascular reactions, both to laboratory tests, like mental arithmetic and TV games, and during their normal working day. As a result, he divided them into *hot responders* who showed exaggerated reactions to challenging, but at the same time normal, everyday events; and *cold responders* who didn't. Although hot responders are more common among Type As, he believes that 'many type B persons show hot reactivity as well'.

He found that large differences existed in heart rate and blood pressure arousal from one person to another, but any one individual's responses were fairly stable. A hot responder is still likely to be hot in six months' time, as David Glass also found. In Eliot's opinion: '. . . physiological testing is the only way to determine the hot reactor. If you know who the hot reactor is and he reports feeling stressed, then one can be confident that his blood pressure will be highly elevated. This is not the case for the cold reactor.' His views coincide with those of Dembroski, who worked with him at one time, when he says that: '. . . a direct measure of challenge-induced physiological response might serve as a predictor of CHD.'

And indeed it might – I would be the last to argue. The problem is who you measure the 'challenge-induced physiological response' on. Surely you don't screen the whole population. Testing sessions are time-consuming, cost money and are certainly not necessary for everyone. Overdrivers are still a minority, even in the United States. Like twenty-four-hour ECG monitoring or coronary angiography, the testing has to be reserved for 'high risk' groups. Perhaps we may look forward to the day when physicians or even general practitioners are able to spot Type As and refer them for testing, just like patients today suspected of having a coronary blockage are referred for an exercise electrocardiogram.

So I'm only one of many who have to disagree when Eliot is reported as saying: 'Forget "type A" as an isolated cause . . . the additional heart attack risk associated with type A behavior is statistically equivalent to failure to buckle your auto safety belts. Many crabby type As have lived to bury their quiet type Bs.'

We don't forget it because it's still the best clue we've got as to who is an overdriver. We don't forget it because the overdriving Type A has special health problems. We don't forget it because he's an unhappy man who we might be able to do something for, and we don't forget it because he's an inefficient worker, and we can certainly do something for that.

No one doubts that Type A is only the *starting point* in the search for those individuals who need testing the most and treating the most. Three-quarters of the Type A men, even in the highest risk group of the WCGS, showed no coronary disease over the eight and a half years that the study was running. What was special about the quarter who did? We may never know. The information was never recorded. The investigators can't be blamed for not asking about factors that hadn't been discovered. But as the years have gone by, risks have emerged that are distinct, not only from blood pressure, cholesterol and the physical risk factors, but distinct from Type A as well.

They are known collectively as 'psychosocial' factors – a psychologist's term for the way that your environment affects your mind, which in its turn affects your body. We have already looked at the control that you are able to exert over your job. But we now turn to a few influences that are rather more personal and that may help decide whether you get a coronary or not.

6. Raising the Odds

How much impact would it make on your life if your wife or husband died? And how much readjustment would it need to get you back into gear after a divorce, after being in gaol, losing your job or taking on a heavy mortgage?

The answer depends partly on your ethnic background. White American men rate bereavement and divorce first and second, ahead of any other of life's disturbances. But black American men rate divorce a long way down, well below the problems of having a big mortgage or going to gaol. For Mexican Americans, marriage is the number one event. Divorce is tenth and going to gaol is only nineteenth on their list.

Why are these ratings important in our thinking about overdrive? Because the number of disturbances that you have in your life and the number of adjustments that you have to make to come to terms with them have a major impact on your health. Of course, this has been suspected for centuries, but serious research to try to prove it started only in the 1950s. Since that time a whole series of studies have linked these 'life changes' with the onset of health problems as diverse as tuberculosis, leukaemia and multiple sclerosis, diabetes, accidents and athletic injuries, to say nothing of psychiatric complaints, sudden death and myocardial infarction.

The first major contribution to the study of life change events was made by Dr Richard H. Rahe of the US Navy Neuropsychiatric Unit in San Diego and the University of

California, Los Angeles. The yardstick that Rahe and others used to establish just how disturbed your life may have been is a 42-item questionnaire known as the Schedule of Recent Experience, or SRE. It is a check-list of possible events that may have happened to you. They range from bereavement, divorce and gaol, through personal injury or illness, retirement, death of a close friend and trouble with your in-laws, to less dramatic disturbances like changing your working hours or living through Christmas.

In its original form, all the events were treated in the same way. You got a point for every one that had occurred in your recent life. But obviously, they don't all affect you to the same extent. Some may be devastating, others almost routine. So it was decided in the early 1960s to put a score on each one, so their impacts could be compared. Groups of people in the USA (and in other countries too) were given the list and told that marriage rated 50 points. They were then asked to rate the others on the basis of how much disruption each would cause. Different groups came up with rather different ratings. But a schedule used widely among white Americans puts the death of a spouse first with 100 points. Divorce has 73, retirement 45, and so on down to Christmas with 12. When all the points that you've gained over a period of months or years are added up, the resulting score is your total of life change units or LCUs.

Even the early work from the mid-1960s found a link between LCU scores and health problems like infection and accidents. People with up to 150 points in any particular year were likely to have good health in the twelve months that followed. Half of those scoring between 150 and 300 would probably have some illness in the following year, and seven out of ten of those scoring more than 300 were destined to suffer, often from multiple bouts of sickness.

So the SRE looked interesting, but it needed a lot more testing. Because of his navy connections, Rahe was able to set up a number of large-scale studies on board ship. In many ways this arrangement was ideal for research. Sailors' past medical histories were all on file, and illnesses other than the most trivial were reported to the ship's doctors who built up a very complete health record of everyone in the ship's company.

In the first investigation, 2500 officers and men, more or less the whole complement of three cruisers, recorded their life change scores for the previous four years. These were broken down into six-monthly periods and compared with the actual illness records for each man in each of these half years. About 1700 of them reported some illness over the period. A year before they became ill, most of those were showing LCU scores of about 100. Six months before, their scores had risen to 125 and in the six months of the illness itself they ran about 175. So there seemed to be a gradual build-up of life changes over a year and a half, culminating in the sickness. This was even more noticeable when they were compared to men who showed no illness in the four years. They had been running scores of only about 85.

A second shipboard study, again on three cruisers, was even more elegant. The men were at sea for a six-month tour of duty and any illnesses that they experienced during the voyage were duly recorded. They were mostly what navy physicians would call 'minor complaints' – digestive upsets, urinary tract and venereal disease, muscular strains and skin problems. When the men's records in the six months before they put to sea were looked at, it was clear that those with the highest life change scores before sailing had reported more illness than those with the lowest. The study was later repeated on 1000 men in the Norwegian navy who were followed for more than a year. The results again showed that as the LCU scores increased, so did the sickness rate.

Now all that's fine for the minor illnesses you might find in a healthy group of men. By the very nature of their jobs, seamen have to be fairly fit. If not, they leave the service. But what about civilians who are less fit; what about women; and what about more serious disease, particularly CHD? Do life changes help to predict that as well?

The pilot study of life events and CHD, a study of sudden cardiac death, was published in 1971. It was another American/Swedish collaboration in which Rahe worked with Evy Lind of the Seraphimer Hospital in Stockholm.

We have seen how sudden death can immediately follow some physical exertion or emotional upheaval. Rahe and Lind also believed that 'the effect of life stress, if any, upon subject's susceptibility to sudden cardiac death, may well take place over a longer time span than just the final few minutes to hours prior to death'. So they set out to discover from the widows or children of thirty-nine sudden death victims in Stockholm, what sort of lives they had in the three years prior to the attack. Obviously, asking the relatives may give a distorted answer. They may not remember things (or choose not to remember them) as they really were.

But even allowing for faulty memories, the results were positive. Sudden death may be the first you know about having CHD, or you may have had warning signs like angina or a previous myocardial infarction. For the ten Swedish victims who had no warning, life event scores had increased in the year before the attack, and in the six months before they increased threefold. With the other twenty-nine deceased, who already had a history of CHD, the rise had started earlier – two and a half years before the attack – and it too had increased right up to the fatal event. So for MI victims, both with symptoms and without, an increased LCU score predicted their deaths.

But what about the survivors of myocardial infarction; do

life events predict their illness too? Rahe studied this question with a number of collaborators, including Dr Töres Theorell, then also at the Seraphimer Hospital. Firstly, they looked at fifty-four infarction survivors who were still in the hospital. They asked them to fill in the SRE for the few years prior to their attack, and also to provide the name of a friend or colleague similar to them in age, but who hadn't had a heart attack. These friends made up a comparison group and so they also filled in the 42-item check-list. The differences between the patients and their friends were very marked. The patients showed a distinct rise in life change events in the two years before the infarction. The friends didn't.

Rahe and his team then turned their attention to infarction victims who had recovered sufficiently to go home. Thirty of them completed the check-list for the four years before their attack. The change in life event scores for each three-month period was quite obvious. Starting at a baseline level of about 20–30, it crept up to more than 50 over the year and a half before the infarction. Interestingly enough, in the year after the attack, it fell back to about 25. Whatever the hassle had been before the illness, it seemed to have disappeared afterwards, in this small group of thirty outpatients at least. But though the researchers didn't say so, the infarction victim who can get the problem out of his life is a lucky man. Others don't, and the result may be a second infarction.

We've concentrated on men, simply because more of them have heart attacks. But sixty-one women with coronaries in Helsinki also showed a similar pattern. Those suffering myocardial infarction or sudden death had a much greater increase in life changes in the six months preceding the attack, than in the same period of the year before.

Richard Rahe once wrote that: 'The life change questionnaire simply documents changes in subjects' on-going adjustments in central areas of concern in their lives.'

How these adjustments show themselves depends more than anything else on *who* is doing the adjusting, but it was just these *individual* responses to life events that seemed at one time to put the whole subject into doubt. In a further study, Töres Theorell, together with Evy Lind and Dr Ulf Lundberg in Stockholm, asked fifty-six MI survivors to record their life changes for the year leading up to the attack, and the 46 items were then rated by a group of healthy Swedes, in terms of how upsetting each would be for them, and how much adjustment it would need to get their lives back to normal afterwards. But the ratings by these healthy people didn't predict infarction among the patients at all.

So Theorell's group asked the patients *themselves* to rate each item, and when the averages of the patients' *own* scores were used, life events predicted illness as usual. The difference in the way that patients and healthy people saw certain events was quite striking. For example, infarction victims gave increased responsibility at work an average score of 48. Healthy people only gave it 25. Again, a change in sexual habits got an average of 53 from the group of patients. Healthy people gave it only 23. And the upset involved in taking on an extra job scored 20 among the patients, but only 2 among those who were fit and well. All of these are changes that healthy people can easily take in their stride. But after an infarction they need a lot of effort.

The Swedish team went one further. Instead of using the average rating for the patients as a group, they also took each individual patient's *own* ratings for the 46 events and related them to the life changes leading up to the infarction. And these personal scales, applied in each individual case, gave the best prediction of all.

So the researchers reached a conclusion that will surprise no one who has stayed with me so far: 'The risk of illness onset for individual subjects should be judged according to the individually perceived life stress.' Remember Friedman's tax accountants? Their cholesterol levels were at a peak on days when *they* thought they were under the greatest pressure. Remember the core beliefs of the Type A? His perception of life as a 'zero sum game' may be a delusion, but for him it's real enough and his body reacts accordingly.

The importance of the personal rating of life events has also been noticed by cardiologists in other countries. Drs D. G. Byrne and H. M. Whyte at the Australian National University in Canberra compared more than a hundred infarction patients, men and women, with a group who had been admitted to the same hospital with chest pains but who later had been found not to have an infarction. Both groups filled out a very full inventory of life events for the twelve months leading up to their hospital admission. In addition, they were asked to judge, for each event, just how much disruption it had caused them at the time it happened, how much adjustment it had taken afterwards and how far it had left them feeling depressed, anxious, angry or helpless.

The MI patients didn't actually have more life changes in the year before the attack than the patients with chest pain, but they did experience more upset, depression and helplessness. At highest risk for myocardial infarction were those who found their life changes in the previous year to be particularly distressing. In other words, infarction patients *feel* that they have suffered more emotional upheaval. There is no sure way of checking back to see whether they actually have, but that hardly matters. It is the victim's *own* assessment that is all-important. So, easily aroused distress caused by unpleasant situations may be an added risk leading to a coronary, particularly for the overdriver. And, of course, he may be largely to blame for bringing it on himself.

The go-getting Type A, constantly trying to compete and produce, always eager to acquire more of everything and to do so faster than last week is going to expose himself to more life changes than the easygoing Type B. He's more likely to change his job, to relocate to another area, and to settle into a new neighbourhood. This puts a strain on him directly. It also put strains on his wife and family that will rebound and affect him too. After half a dozen different addresses his wife may be reluctant to move yet again; after several changes of school, his children may fall so far behind that they give up trying, and this is guaranteed to infuriate their father, who never gave up trying in his life. And so the Type A adds to his problem by seeking change, even though he may genuinely believe that he thrives on the challenge.

There's also another side to the problem. Many people who are only moderately Type A find themselves having a difficult time every now and again. Many of us have lived through a period when the workload is high and promotion is a real possibility, but time to complete the project is short. In these circumstances, even a Type X may take on an increasingly Type A persona, just to get the job done and keep his time-wasting colleagues out of his hair until the assignment is completed. Unfortunately, gearing down again is not so easy once you've tasted the short-term success that Type A can bring. He may find himself easier to arouse on the next occasion. So he's in danger of becoming an A1 by degrees.

Whichever way it happens, the overdriver who has gone through a distressing series of life events in the past year or two is likely to be a higher coronary risk than someone who hasn't. The effect may not be immediate. Changes occurring over a couple of years, and particularly those that take place in the last three to six months, seem to have the biggest impact.

But what turns life events into pathology?

Theorell, Lind and others reasoned that if catecholamines increase in response to new situations, then life events, which are generally unexpected, should make them rise as well. To test the idea they looked at a group of twenty-one rehabilitated infarction patients, men in their mid-fifties, who had been discharged from hospital and who were living at home. They were asked to record all the significant events that occurred in their lives over a period of five months, and every couple of weeks they went back to the hospital to have urine samples taken for catecholamine levels.

Some weeks, when they sat down with the interviewer, they had little to report. At other times their lives had been quite eventful. The most common problems were conflict at home and at work, changes in work patterns and the distress of having to stay at home because of illness. For example, one fifty-seven-year-old tailor admitted to a series of arguments and irritations at work during the first week of the study. In weeks two and three he had to stay home because his face was paralysed. He went back to work in week four and the following week he spent a lot of time arranging the apartment for his son to come and live with them. In week six he had such a blazing row with his boss that he tried to kill himself and he spent the next two weeks in a mental ward. In week nine nothing happened, and in week ten his wife became seriously ill.

This Swedish tailor is hardly typical, as most people don't pack so many life events into two and a half months. But he shows very well the ups and downs, from weeks of distress to weeks of comparative calm. Theorell found that during the weeks with no significant life changes, urinary catecholamine levels were below average. In contrast, during weeks with important changes, the volunteers' adrenaline and noradrenaline levels both rose and followed their life change scores.

So life events, or at least the way we see our changing life events, may raise our catecholamines, with all that entails. The more changes we have, and the more distressing we find them, the greater the increase is likely to be. So we might search for high risk coronary subjects, either by giving them a Schedule of Recent Experience to fill in, or by measuring the catecholamines in their blood or urine.

Another way is to look at their mood and morale. Psychologists have recently been doing just that – looking for the emotional changes that go with illness. What they're searching for are any outward signs that will identify individuals in risk groups so high that they need emergency attention.

David Jenkins made a detailed study of the connection between what he calls 'sustained disturbing emotions' and heart disease. The most obvious of these emotions are anxiety and depression, disturbances that we all suffer from at some time in our lives. Most of us get over them, but Jenkins has collected together studies from centres as far apart as Israel, Scandinavia and the United States, showing that for some people they may have more serious consequences. In susceptible individuals, both anxiety and depression seem related to angina and coronary death. The emotional disturbances that best predict infarction are a feeling of being drained and exhausted, and difficulty in getting enough sleep.

Jenkins's own group in Boston looked at sleep problems as part of a large-scale study of men who were waiting for coronary bypass surgery. Interested in the psychological problems that such patients face, Jenkins and his colleagues interviewed more than a hundred of them. Obviously, they weren't able to study infarction. The whole point of the surgery was to stop an infarction from happening. But they did look at angina, the symptom that had brought most of the men to the hospital in the first place. Angina can be brought on both by exertion and emotion, and the Boston group found that sleep problems were one of the best predictors of both.

Is that cause or effect? Does the heart patient's anxiety or depression bring on the attack, or are the victims depressed because they know they have heart disease? Usually we have no way of knowing, but sometimes we do. Future heart patients may be examined *before* the disease shows itself, and when this happens there is no doubt that emotional disturbances often come first. Dr W. H. Orchard of the Australian National Heart Foundation found that 70–80 per cent of those patients who are destined to suffer from the effects of heart disease are already in a state of 'masked depression' before the disease appears. It remains masked simply because they continue with their pattern of frantic activity. Many doctors don't recognize it, and the patients usually deny it as well. For most of them it is the first period of serious depression that they have had in their lives and it takes a lot of persuasion even to get them to admit that it is happening.

What does it feel like? Victims describe it as a state of fatigue, exhaustion or helplessness. They lose interest in their work and in their home lives. Nothing seems to have any point any more. As one of them put it: 'Whatever I do, something seems to crop up to wipe it out.' Some of the most detailed studies of the emotional problems of future heart patients have been done in the Netherlands by Professor Ad Appels and Dr Paul Falger who work at the School of Medicine at the State University of Limburg. Both of them were struck by the fact that perhaps as many as seven out of every ten future victims of infarction or sudden coronary death go to their doctor in the year before the attack. The majority of them complain of chest pain, but many also say that they feel weak or fatigued.

The Dutch group produced a questionnaire of their own, designed to get at what the future heart patient was actually feeling – was he tired, anxious, depressed? The town where much of this research was done is called Maastricht, and so the form that they devised was called the Maastricht Questionnaire or MQ. In their early studies they gave it to nearly four hundred patients who had visited their family doctor complaining of cardiac symptoms. Then they followed these patients up for about a year, looking for the appearance of any new coronary event, like MI or sudden death. They found that patients who did develop new coronary disease had high MQ scores when they went to see the doctor in the first place. They experienced a particular cluster of feelings, including exhaustion and lack of vitality, depression and a hypochondriac concern with their bodies.

The next stage was to compare the MQ results from a group of fifty-eight patients who had already had one infarction with scores from a similar number of healthy people. Would the MQ score distinguish between them? It did. Indeed, it did so better than the patient's Type A or B status, which was measured at the same time using the structured interview. Falger and Appels think that exhaustion and depression might be better indicators simply because they happen closer to the time of the infarction than any part of Type A, which has more to do with the way that the victim has been behaving for years.

But surely these distressing emotions and the patient's Type A make-up interact in some way? And where do life changes come in all this? To study these questions they took 136 healthy young men and had them all complete the Maastricht Questionnaire. They also gave them the Jenkins Activity Survey and another form, similar to the Schedule of Recent Experience, that had questions about life changes in the last two years, both at home and at work. They predicted that the 70 Type As in this group would have had more distressing life changes in the recent past than the 66 Type

Bs. And they were right. Type As had more serious marital problems as well as more work problems, both with supervisors and subordinates.

Their second prediction was that those men who were particularly exhausted and depressed on the MQ scale would have suffered more distressing life changes during the previous two years than those with lower MQ scores. Again they were right. Men who found themselves most often exhausted also had more problems with their children and conflicts with their wives, as well as more financial troubles. And they had experienced all these changes over a shorter period than men scoring lower on the MQ. Finally, they found that, as a group, Type As also had higher MQ scores. So life changes, exhaustion and Type A go together.

Even so, Type A and loss of vitality are *independent* predictors of infarction, and so anyone unfortunate enough to score high on both the JAS and the MQ is like a cigarette smoker with high blood pressure. He has two risk factors that interact and one risk multiplies the other. We don't know whether distressing life events are a third independent predictor. They may simply lead to the feeling of helplessness that the MQ measures. But the Type A who feels helpless and depressed because of events in his recent past must be in an especially high-risk bracket. These may have been just the men who didn't survive to the end of the WCGS.

Where do these disturbing emotions come from? What makes men answer 'yes' to questionnaire items about depression ('Do you sometimes wish to be dead?'), exhaustion ('Do you sometimes have the feeling that your body is a battery that is losing its power?') and not being able to cope ('Do you have the feeling that the younger people are trying to push out the older ones?'). They may inevitably result from reaching a certain age, a certain stage in your career and your life cycle.

But the Maastricht team have other ideas. Their own explanation is based on David Glass's idea of swinging between hyperactivity and hypoactivity. Being hyperactive may be exhausting, but at least it gets things done. It's hypoactivity that takes over when you feel that your efforts aren't producing any results. Appels and Falger believe that this pattern can slowly creep up on you. Every time you have a failure, it makes the chance of you failing again (or at least, of behaving as though you had) just that little bit greater. After this has happened many times you gradually begin to get used to failing. The pattern starts to become ingrained, just as hyperactivity did earlier in your life. Eventually, you may stop trying altogether, and take refuge in your exhaustion. They don't call it 'burn-out', but what they are describing comes pretty close – slow retreat into yourself and away from a world that is getting increasingly more difficult to cope with.

But that doesn't explain why the failures start in the first place. After all, only a minority of men slide downhill like this. Perhaps those who do are the ones with advancing atheroma. Maybe performing at the rate they did ten or twenty years ago really does need an immense amount of effort. Maybe, as their CAD creeps on, they simply can't perform as well as they used to, or maybe they just let themselves think they can't.

In the 1970s a most revealing heart disease study was conducted in south-eastern Connecticut and the results were reported by Drs Walter I. Wardwell and C. B. Bahnson. They compared 114 MI survivors with a similar number of people hospitalized for other disorders, and with a group of normal people. They were looking for differences between them that might predict heart disease in the future and they found a couple. The first was a measure of Type A behaviour, arrived at through an assessment scale of their own. Nothing surprising there.

But the second was more unexpected. It was described as 'somatization' – a tendency for people to translate the conflicts that they find in their environment into symptoms in their own bodies. Recall that Falger and Appels also found a hypochondriac streak in their high MQ scorers. The MI patients in Connecticut said that they often felt nauseous, got indigestion and severe colds, and felt tired a good deal of the time. So struck were the two investigators by this pattern that they even suggested that: '. . . what counts in the production of MI may not be the amount of situational or intrapsychic stress a person is subjected to, but the way he copes with it, his defensive style.' So we're back to the individual with his own particular way of facing the world.

But though we have to save our own lives, we need other people too. Nobody's act is a solo. Many overdrivers realize this too late. For Irving, the rediscovery of his wife and son only happened in intensive care, and others aren't even that lucky. Years of hurry and hostility have cut them off from the support that might keep them alive. The overdriver who thinks no one cares about him may well be right. And he probably got there entirely by his own efforts.

Typical of what I mean are a group of fifty infarction patients who were admitted to hospital at the Oklahoma School of Medicine in the early 1970s. The men, all aged between forty and sixty, were a cross-section of American overdrive. Many of them had two full-time jobs, and some worked for more than seventy hours a week. The champion was a truck-driver who worked twelve to sixteen hours almost every day. Following the research programme that we have now seen so often, these patients were matched with fifty healthy subjects who resembled them closely, apart from the MI. The two groups then went through a battery of tests to see if the comparison would show up anything about the patients that might have caused their heart attacks.

Obviously, the number of hours they worked each day was one difference between them. But there were plenty of others as well. Everyone filled in an anxiety questionnaire ('Do you get upset easily?' 'Do you often feel restless and tense?') and the MI patients got the highest average. There was a similar questionnaire for depression, where they were asked if statements like 'I get tired for no reason', 'I feel useless' and 'Every day seems exactly the same' would apply to them. And the statements did apply, far more often than they applied to the healthy volunteers.

The questionnaire also looked at their family circumstances, where even bigger differences started to emerge. For example, 36 per cent of the patients had been divorced, three times more than the healthy men. One in seven said that he often felt lonely, while only one in fifty of the healthy group did, and the infarction victims were nearly three times as likely to have lost friends in recent years.

So the picture that emerges is of an MI victim who is not only an anxious and depressed workaholic, but also feels isolated and lonely, and the results of bigger surveys show the same. The National Center for Disease Statistics published an analysis of CHD patterns among some seven thousand US citizens (taken incidentally from one of the same surveys that Karasek used to look at job pressures and health). They found that coronary death rates among both men and women who were divorced, widowed or who had never married were higher than those in married people. A team at Johns Hopkins also examined the death rate among a thousand men and three thousand women in Maryland who had lost their wives or husbands between 1963 and 1974. Widowhood didn't have much effect on the death rate of women, but among widowers between eighteen and forty-four, the death rate from all causes was nearly three times higher than for men whose wives were still alive.

Interestingly enough, if widowers remarried, their

mortality rates came down again. When Dr Samuel Johnson, the compiler of the first English dictionary, described second marriage as 'the triumph of hope over experience' he obviously didn't have access to the mortality figures. So impressive are these statistics that one British university teacher, asked by a student what he could do to prevent a heart attack replied without hesitation, 'Stop smoking and get yourself a wife.'

But it's not just marriage that gives you protection. The same study showed that both men and women living alone had higher mortality rates than those living with someone else. Just having someone in the house increases your chance of survival. There's nothing mysterious about that. With someone to keep an eye on you there's less chance of you injuring yourself, either deliberately or by accident, and more chance of your eating properly and getting to bed at night. So at one level 'social support' just means protecting you from yourself.

But it means much more than that. Professor Sidney Cobb of Brown University in Rhode Island has described how social support acts at several different levels. First is the type of support that assures the subject that he is cared for and loved – very much that provided by a wife and family. Then comes the support that assures him he is esteemed and valued at his workplace or in his neighbourhood. And related to that is the support that he gets from the feeling that he belongs to a 'network' – a larger group of people with shared interests or beliefs. Cobb concluded that 'adequate social support can protect people in crisis from a wide variety of pathological states from low birth weight to death, from arthritis through tuberculosis to depression, alcoholism and other psychiatric illness'.

As an example, let's pick up on the last of these – psychiatric illness. And to keep things simple, let's look first at people who you might expect to be particularly supportive to each other – a minority ethnic group. With this in mind, Dr Nan Lin and colleagues decided to examine the mental health of a group of men and women of Chinese origin in Washington DC by asking them how often they felt sad, depressed or otherwise mentally disturbed. Their replies were matched with the answers that they gave to other questionnaire items about how involved they were with the Chinese community. They were asked how often they got together with friends from the old country, how frequently they talked to their neighbours and so on.

Though the end-points were rather crude, the results were clear enough. Individuals high on social support had fewer symptoms of mental disturbance. It was the same message as came from Detroit. There may not be much you can do about the distressing events in your life. But there is a good deal you can do to plug into the social networks around you. And the reward is well worth the effort.

A wider investigation, from Alameda County, California, points in exactly the same way. In 1965 Professor S. Leonard Syme from Berkeley together with Dr Lisa F. Berkman from Yale supervised a large-scale project in which enumerators went round to over four thousand households in the County. They collected answers from nearly seven thousand adults about their family and friendship ties as well as about a whole variety of health practices. These people were then followed up until 1974, and it says a lot for the organization of the project that during those nine years only 4 per cent of them lost contact with the study.

The object was to discover what effect social support had on mortality. The support itself was seen as coming from four sources, marriage, contact with close friends and relatives, churchgoing and group associations. Each source conferred some protection. So unmarried men between thirty and forty-nine were three times more likely to die than married men, confirming what we have already seen. The other sources of support were not as strongly protective, but even people regularly attending a church or temple had lower death rates than those who didn't. Since each type of support acted independently of the others, Berkman and Syme were able to produce an overall support measure, taking all these sources into account and making adjustments for their relative importance. Low scores on this measure were associated with increased heart disease, cancer, stroke and other causes of death.

Now, we have to keep our sense of proportion. Alameda County must be one of the most affluent areas anywhere on the globe, and six inhabitants out of ten had a low mortality risk. Only when there was increasing social disconnection did the death rate start to rise sharply. Even so, those men who took care of their health by following a few simple health practices and who were also well supported, were five times less likely to die than those who didn't and weren't. For women too this combination of elementary health care, together with a wide social network, conferred a threefold protection. And anyone who turns their back on a 300–500 per cent better chance of staying alive really is in need of help.

Social support protects against such a wide range of diseases that there must be many pathways leading from isolation to illness. But anyone looking for some general pattern can find one, and by now it comes as no surprise. Listen to Berkman and Syme's own suggestion: '. . . the central role psychosocial factors play in the causation of disease is not due to the stressful objective circumstances, but to the way in which these circumstances are more subjectively perceived and mediated by the individual.'

And should you need an even bigger demonstration of the same thing, let's finally look at some work done in Israel by Professor J. H. Medalie, who subsequently came to work at Case Western Reserve in Cleveland. Medalie and his colleagues followed the development of infarction and angina in no less than ten thousand Israeli government and municipal employees in the mid-1960s. They discovered a number of disease predictors. For example, higher infarction rates occurred among men who thought their superiors didn't appreciate the work they were doing. Sounds familiar? On the other hand, they found lower rates of infarction among religious men and among those who received love and support from their wives.

The results for angina are even more interesting than those for infarction. Among a host of possible risk factors that they examined, seven were found to predict chest pain developing over the next five years. They were advancing age, high cholesterol, high blood pressure, an abnormal ECG, diabetes, anxiety and a cluster of psychosocial problems. Among the latter, family difficulties were particularly important, though again the perception was relative. The sort of family trouble described as 'serious' by various men ranged from the rebellion of an adolescent daughter or the need to cope with a backward son, to not having his dinner on the table when he came home. But whatever the provocation to angina, having a loving and supportive wife reduced it.

Why was anxiety a risk factor for chest pain? The Israeli team suggested that it was boosting the release of cortisol and catecholamines. But with someone to share the hassle, the anginal sufferer could keep his arousal down to a level where he could handle it.

And that's precisely what we want to do for the overdriver – to stop his exaggerated reactions from taking off. The higher his risk the more important it becomes to teach him how to make sense of his environment, how to tell what's important from what isn't, and how to act accordingly. That's what I mean by a 'flexible response'. The greater his overdriving compulsion, the more important it also becomes to teach him how to listen to his body and its signs of distress.

Can we do these things? We can do some of them, and now we're going to look at how. We've heard quite enough about death. The second half of this book is about life – your life – and what *you* can do to save it.

7. Cholesterol Revisited

The research centre that has had more to do with coronary disease in the last twenty years than any other in the world is a branch of the National Institutes of Health in Bethesda, Maryland. It has had several names in its time, but it is currently known as the National Heart, Lung and Blood Institute, or NHLBI. At the end of the 1970s, when Dr Robert I. Levy was its director, he had a huge cartoon hanging over his office door. The scene was a round-table conference of high-ranking physicians. The doctor addressing them (perhaps Levy himself) was holding up a copy of the *New York Times* that carried a banner headline: 'Twenty per cent fall in US heart disease deaths.' 'Gentlemen,' he was saying to them, 'I have called you here to try to decide what we're doing right.'

The cartoon marked the discovery that between 1968 and 1977 the death rate from coronary disease had fallen in the USA. Some two hundred thousand fewer deaths had occurred than anyone could have predicted on the basis of the trends in the 1960s. Coronary death rates had also been falling in a few other countries, like Canada, Australia and Belgium. But in the rest of the world, including the United Kingdom, they had been steady, or actually rising. The American fall was certainly more dramatic than anywhere else.

No one knew why, and it has still not been established, although everyone has their own opinion. In an attempt to get an answer the NHLBI called together an expert panel in

October 1978. First, was the fall in mortality real, or was it simply the result of changing the way that deaths were recorded over the years? Everyone agreed that the change was real. The important question was whether heart attack victims were being kept alive better, or whether fewer people were actually getting the disease.

Certainly, ambulances were faster, paramedics better trained, monitoring and surgery more advanced, and rehabilitation more effective than they had been in the 1960s. But you would have to be a real optimist to believe that the change was entirely due to better medical care. The death rate among hospital coronary patients had fallen – but only by 10 per cent – and seven out of ten of them were dead before they got there.

So was the attack rate falling; were people finally heeding the statistics and acting on them – smoking less, eating their prudent diets and running their ten or twenty miles a week? One of the best-known experts in preventive medicine, Professor Jeremiah Stamler of the Northwestern University Medical School in Chicago, showed how a fall of only 5 per cent in the average level of cholesterol in the blood of American men would account for a quarter of the fall in the coronary death rate. An even smaller reduction in blood pressure would explain another quarter, and a 15 per cent decline in cigarette smoking among middle-aged men would account for the other half. So, as he says: '. . . the data do fit. They certainly are consistent with – and lend support to – the hypothesis that reduced mortality rates are a result of changes in risk factor status in the population.'

It's tempting to believe that he is right. But it's not that easy. Firstly, it is not clear whether the rate of non-fatal attacks has actually changed at all. The NHLBI, in their carefully worded summary of the conference, admit as much: '. . . a precise quantification of the causes requires further studies, especially those designed to document whether the frequency of nonfatal coronary events is changing.'

Then again, it is immensely difficult to discover whether risk factors have changed either. For every trend, the panel lists a counter-trend. Though no one doubts that Americans in the 1970s ate fewer eggs and less butter than in the previous decade, total fat and meat consumption actually showed an increase. Any resulting effect on the level of cholesterol in the nation's blood serum must have been small.

During the 1970s, high blood pressure started to be sought out and treated, as physicians say, 'aggressively'. But treatment was still confined to the one person in ten or twenty with the highest blood pressure levels, and such treatment, however aggressive, can have had little influence on the average blood pressure of Americans as a whole.

Then there's smoking. The tar and nicotine content of cigarettes has fallen since the mid-1960s, as has the number of smokers. But it seems that the proportion of heavy smokers, i.e., those who smoke two or more packs a day, hasn't changed, and while smoking has fallen most among men, heart disease deaths have fallen fastest among women. Exercise too has become enormously popular, but only among particular sections of the American public. According to the NHLBI, 'its effect on a decline in mortality beginning in the mid-1960s must be minimal'.

Finally, there's the embarrassing fact that by making a few quite reasonable assumptions you can explain not only the fall that actually occurred but more or less any fall you like. As one specialist remarked, perhaps a little tongue in cheek, if everyone's favourite risk factor accounted for just 15 per cent of the decline, then putting them all together would explain a drop in mortality ten times greater than the one that has actually taken place.

Professor Lester Bristow, Dean of the School of Public Health at the University of California in Los Angeles, pointed out to the NHLBI meeting that the American death rate from *all causes* reached a plateau in the mid-1950s. This was because earlier killers like tuberculosis, pneumonia and influenza had largely been brought under control, while coronary disease and lung cancer continued to rise. After a decade with little change, the trend turned downwards again, with heart deaths falling at a rate of more than 2 per cent every year. But this fall in coronary deaths only accounts for two lives saved out of every five. Cancers (apart from cancer of the lung) and deaths from stroke were also declining, so rather than concentrating just on coronaries, we should see the falling number of heart deaths as part of a more general pattern of mortality improvement in the United States. As Bristow says, 'The drop in mortality may have been influenced by factors that extend beyond a specific category of disease.'

We have already seen an example of some of the factors that he had in mind. They are the seven health practices put forward by Lisa Berkman and Leonard Syme, in Alameda County, California, and before that by Dr Nedra Belloc of the California State Department of Public Health. They are not smoking; taking regular exercise; maintaining your weight within a certain range for your height; drinking moderately; eating breakfast; not eating between meals; and sleeping seven to eight hours a night. The whole package is not so much a formula for reducing coronary risks as a guide to sensible living, and it works remarkably well.

I have already described how a hefty 23-page questionnaire was given to nearly seven thousand people in Alameda County in early 1975. It contained questions about their medical history, family life, education and income. Five years later the same subjects were followed up to assess the effect of their living habits on their subsequent survival.

Men and women who never smoked had a lower risk of dying over the five years than those who did. And men who took part in active sport had only half the mortality rate of those who exercised only rarely. Then there was the question of weight. There are many published tables showing the average weight for a given height that may be found among large groups of people. But the average doesn't necessarily mean the most healthy. Indeed, the mortality rate in Alameda County was lowest, not for those men of average weight, but for those who were 10–19 per cent over it. Those under the average had a greater chance of dying, as did those with a weight excess of 20 per cent or more.

Moderate drinking, one or two drinks at a sitting, seemed to give better protection than drinking either more or less, and having a regular breakfast and not eating between meals were independent ways of lowering the risk. As to sleep, eight hours was the healthiest figure for men, six or seven for women.

Now there are some reservations about these figures and the Californian workers were quick to admit them. Sometimes it isn't possible to unravel cause from effect. For example, men who don't exercise may simply be too ill to do so; women who sleep only five hours a night may have deep-seated anxieties that keep them awake. So when we consider the value of a healthy lifestyle we have to allow for such things as illness or anxiety biasing the figures. Then again, the protection may not be the same for other groups of people living different lives in other parts of the world. For them the risks aren't the same either.

But even with these provisos, the gains are impressive. Nedra Belloc calculated that a man of forty-five who followed three or fewer of these health practices could expect to live until he was sixty-seven. But for the man practising six or seven, his expectation was raised to an age of seventy-eight, a net gain of eleven years, or nearly four times the natural increase in life span that had occurred among American men since 1900. For women following all these practices the gain was seven years, not quite so impressive perhaps, but then American women can expect to live seven years longer than men anyway.

Berkman and Syme extended these studies in Alameda County from five up to nine years, and they found that, other things being equal, both men and women pursuing six or seven of these healthy practices had only half the death rate of those with four or less. But of course other things never are equal. Statisticians only equalize them to make comparisons easier. One particularly unequal feature in Alameda County was the subjects' level of social support – the number of connections they had with various social networks. And when this support was also taken into account, the differences in mortality were amazing. Men aged between thirty and sixty-nine with the maximum amount of social support and six or seven healthy practices were five times more likely to survive over the nine years than those with the least support and least healthy lifestyle. For women, the protection given by social support and lifestyle together was threefold.

So the very simplest way for an overdriver (or anyone else) to increase his chance of surviving is to plug into the social networks around him and adopt a few quite elementary habits (remember 'Stop smoking and get yourself a wife'?).

Unfortunately, many overdrivers feel that they can't. The networks aren't there any more. Most of their family has grown up, gone away or died. And it's so long since they took part in any group activity outside their work that they don't feel they can ever start again.

They're wrong about the last part, as we shall see. Group sessions for overdrivers will be a growth industry in the late 1980s. They can start to change their health practices too. It's really not that difficult to start doing something about the 'standard' risks that their physicians are always warning them about – cholesterol and high blood pressure, cigarettes and inactivity.

The original suggestions that raised cholesterol and blood pressure cause heart disease were made well before World War II. Doubts about smoking and inactivity came later. But large-scale efforts to measure these risk factors – to put numbers on them – only started after the war, and projects began in several places at much the same time. In the spring of 1950, examinations began on some five thousand volunteers in Framingham, Massachusetts. The Framingham Study lasted for twenty-four years, long enough to examine the children of the original volunteers. Similar investigations started in Los Angeles in 1949, Chicago and Albany in the early 1950s and Tecumseh, Michigan, in 1959. Each one confirmed the link between coronary disease and cholesterol, and most found a link with high blood pressure as well.

It became clear in the 1960s that none of these studies was large enough on its own to provide all the information that was needed. So five of them were combined and three others examined in parallel, to give results on a total of over twelve thousand subjects – mostly men and mostly white. The combined study, which became known as the US National Pooling Project, made it possible to examine coronary risks in some detail.

The simplest way into the mountain of figures that the Pooling Project produced is to compare the death rates of men with the highest and lowest risk. Men smoking more than a pack of cigarettes a day are three times more likely to suffer infarction or death than those who don't smoke at all. Those with the highest levels of serum cholesterol have two and a half times the chance of suffering as a result, and those with the highest blood pressures have about twice the risk of those with the lowest. These hazards multiply together, so that if you had the highest level of all three, your risk would be nearly nine times as great as someone with the three lowest. The Pooling Project risk levels were fairly modest, and there are many Americans walking about today in a far worse condition.

None of these risk factors is actually a disease, so why are they dangerous? Let's look first at cholesterol. Although we have come to think of cholesterol as some sort of poison, it's actually an essential part of our bodies, and although it occurs in large quantities in atheroma, a plaque is not simply a bag of grease. Even so, there's no escaping the fact that raised levels of cholesterol in the blood serum go with an increased risk of CHD.

If we compare societies which have a lot of coronary disease, like Finland or Scotland, with those where CHD is rare, as for instance among the Japanese or the Masai tribesmen in Kenya, we find that cholesterol levels are higher in regions where the disease is common. White American men, for example, have an average of somewhere between 190 and 230 milligrams (mg) of cholesterol in each 100 millilitres (ml) of their blood. Southern Japanese have nearer 130. And the annual coronary rate in the USA is more than three times that in Japan.

We can look at wholly American communities like Framingham or Tecumseh and come up with a similar result. The Pooling Project did just that. If you are a white American male, even a non-smoker with low blood pressure, your risk of having your first attack within eight years is twice as high with a cholesterol of 300 as with one of only 200. Cholesterol levels above 220 are bad news, and the higher they go, the worse the news gets.

Your body can make its own cholesterol, but in the West we take a good deal of it in with our food, and you would have to have lived in solitary confinement for the last thirty years not to have heard that eggs and saturated fats (which largely means animal fats) can increase the level of cholesterol in your blood. Even so, some specialists believe that the dangers of dietary fat and cholesterol have been exaggerated.

The rate that your body handles and gets rid of it may be more important than the rate at which you take it in. An average egg contains perhaps 300 mg, and many health diets call for a daily intake far less than that, but when a group of 120 American volunteers (financed it is true by an egg producer) added one egg to their normal food every day for three months, their serum cholesterol showed no particular change. A group of Japanese egg farmers ate up to ten eggs a day to prove the same point. Their serum levels did not rise significantly either.

Of course, you may say, the Japanese are different. But actually we're all different so far as cholesterol is concerned. In a very careful trial in London, fifty-seven volunteers were given about five eggs-worth of cholesterol every day for two weeks. It certainly raised their serum levels, by an average of 29 mg/100 ml. But this average concealed a huge difference between people. The most susceptible had a rise of 75 mg; the least susceptible actually showed a fall.

Despite these different responses, the original thinking behind all low-fat diets was the assumption that lowering serum cholesterol by lowering dietary fat would also lower the coronary rate. It comes as a surprise to many of us, after years of publicity about the evils of animal fats, to learn that no single trial (at least none without serious drawbacks) has ever shown that using diet to lower serum cholesterol among normal people also reduces their death rate. Not only that, but no trial probably ever will show it.

The reason, in a word, is money. Although no one doubts that coronary disease is the number one killer of British and American men, we also have to realize that even in the high cholesterol group, only one in a hundred is likely to have a fatal coronary attack in the next twelve months. To discover whether a change of diet will lower the attack rate we would need a project involving an enormous number of people – perhaps a hundred thousand, according to a feasibility study carried out in the late 1960s. The cost, even then, was estimated at more than half a billion dollars. As long ago as 1971, a Special Task Force on Atherosclerosis called by the National Institutes of Health concluded that 'such a study is not feasible at the present time', and it has certainly become no more feasible in the interim. For example, the recently publicized US Lipid Clinics Trial showed a fall in coronary rates in men with cholesterol levels above 264 treated with the drug *cholestyramine*. It never tried to address the question of what diet does on its own.

Many risk factor trials have tried to maximize their impact by altering a number of risks at once. For example, some twelve hundred men in Oslo were given dietary advice to lower their serum cholesterol and also encouraged to give up smoking. By the end of five years the group who had changed their habits had about half as many infarctions as the group who hadn't. But the specialists running the study admitted that the dietary change on its own wouldn't have produced such a favourable result.

A much larger study was launched by the US Department of Health in 1970. Called the Multiple Risk Factor Intervention Trial (Mr Fit to its friends), it aimed to alter diet, smoking and blood pressure all at the same time, in nearly thirteen thousand high risk men. After seven years of treatment the results were a major disappointment. Risk factors had indeed come down, but there was no difference in mortality between the men simply treated by their own physicians and those receiving an intensive counselling programme. Some optimists suggest that both groups got major benefits, hence the lack of any difference between them. Pessimists say that this is the last time that a budget estimated at $120 million will be spent on this type of research. We may well have seen the last of the big intervention trials.

One thing that such trials have shown is that the fall in

cholesterol achieved in people going about their everyday lives is usually quite small – maybe 10 per cent. Only hospital patients or highly motivated volunteers do much better. Twelve Trappist monks in Belgium lived on a diet reduced in fat and rich in vegetable protein and fibre, and it brought their serum cholesterol down by nearly 30 per cent. But in the world outside the hospital or the monastery, few people are prepared to change their eating to that extent.

In 1964 a European research group started to study the effect of a cholesterol-lowering drug called *clofibrate*. After five years it had reduced the non-fatal infarctions by a quarter, despite the fact that the average fall in cholesterol had been less than 10 per cent. But unfortunately there was also a rise in the total death rate. Other trials have produced similar findings, and it now seems that one of the effects of lowering cholesterol may be to increase the risk of intestinal cancer. At present, health experts are not sure what to make of this apparent link. Many of them point out that the cancer risk is only seen when cholesterol levels reach 190 mg/100 ml or less. Heart disease takes off at about 230, so they recommend us not to panic and keep on taking the diet. Even so, the link has certainly caused a re-think among specialists who once recommended an 'ideal' serum level for the whole American population below 200.

Then what about the much-publicized switch from saturated (animal) to unsaturated (largely vegetable) fats, the basis of the war between butter and margarine? In the 1950s, polyunsaturated fats were thought to protect you against atheroma. Today we're not so sure. Although some unsaturated fats do apparently lower serum cholesterol and prevent thrombosis, the case for deliberately switching to unsaturates isn't yet convincing. They may have problems of their own and advertisers still have to prove their claim that margarine is good for your heart.

So what is a healthy cholesterol level, and when should you

start trying to get yours down? One answer comes from the Pooling Project. Professor Michael Oliver of the University of Edinburgh has recently re-examined the figures. He believes that above the age of forty-five there is no real advantage in reducing your serum cholesterol below 218 mg/ 100 ml. Even if you're younger, there's no benefit in bringing it lower than 195. If your cholesterol is higher then your coronary risk is higher as well. But the increase is gradual at first, and many physicians wouldn't advise you about it until it passed, say, 250. Then they'd advise you to change your diet.

A US Senate Select Committee on Nutrition and Human Needs produced a set of *Dietary Goals for the United States* in 1977, and the American Heart Association Committee on Nutrition endorsed them the following year. Similar recommendations have been made in the UK. 'Not scientifically sound . . . a political and moralistic document . . .' was the reaction of one nutritional expert. What he was objecting to was the recommendation that *everyone* should reduce their fat intake to 30 per cent of their daily calories, bring down their saturated fat to 10 per cent and reduce their daily cholesterol to 300 mg. Housewives wondered how you got from a set of guidelines about saturated fat ratios to a real meal, and the question produced a whole generation of cook books. Christopher Robbins of the British Coronary Prevention Group and Caroline Walker of the Dunn Clinical Nutrition Centre at Cambridge, are just two of the many specialists who have suggested how simple dietary measures, like using skimmed milk instead of whole milk and eating fish and poultry instead of beef and mutton, will reduce the saturated fat content of our diet quite appreciably. Using corn oil for lard gets the saturated content down further. It also puts the proportion of unsaturated fats up, as does the use of vegetable oil for salad dressing. Add to this an increased consumption of fruit, vegetables and cereal fibre and you are getting close to the Senate Committee's recommendations.

The question is whether it's worth doing. It certainly isn't necessary for everybody, and it may not work for everybody either. We have already seen how people vary in their cholesterol response. For those of you who think (or whose doctors think) that you have a problem, then the 'prudent diet' is worth a try. But think of it simply as a way of eating, not a 'medical diet'. It doesn't have to dominate your life.

Of course, there's another side to the cholesterol story that has nothing to do with what you eat. At about the time that the first risk factor studies were getting under way, fifty-five men were volunteering for a quite different type of experiment. They lay in a bath of water at 9°C (48°F, not unbearably cold) for ten minutes. Their serum cholesterols rose by 10 per cent. More familiar with cold water are the US Navy diving and demolition experts that Richard Rahe studied. These specially picked recruits undergo an intensive physical training to get them used to the idea of jumping out of helicopters into the sea. One week of the training is so exhausting that the divers themselves call it 'hell week'. During that week, the serum cholesterol of these fit, super-healthy young men, who had low levels at the beginning, went up, and stayed high for the two weeks that followed.

Less gruelling ordeals can produce similar results. Medical students in Los Angeles had a cholesterol rise of 11 per cent at examination time, and Johns Hopkins students showed a similar increase during their first week settling into medical school, before the examinations were even set. Their patients do worse. Cholesterol levels in people awaiting surgery in hospital have been found to rise by a third or even a half as much as normal. ('A simple, useful guide in assessment of stress,' say the physicians who collected the blood. They don't say what the patients thought about it.)

Distress needn't involve a week of exhaustion or the prospect of going under the knife. Rahe's research team who looked at the navy divers also turned their attention to the investigators themselves. They measured changes in cholesterol as these scientists went about their daily lives. Periods of anxiety, failure or depression sent it up. One of the group spent three months negotiating to buy a house. The deal was on, then off, then on again, and his cholesterol changed more than 50 mg/100 ml during this time. The problem of having nothing to do can produce just the same effect. The experience of your job suddenly closing down under you can cause a whole set of reactions, of which raised cholesterol is just one.

But some recent research shows that cholesterol isn't all bad. It circulates in your blood stream combined with other substances. Two particular combinations are known as low and high density lipoproteins, LDL and HDL. While LDL carries cholesterol into the tissues, so accelerating the rate of atheroma, HDL seems to carry it out again and acts as a protection. Any attempt to lower cholesterol should try to reduce LDL but maintain or even increase the HDL fraction.

Some dietary changes seem to do so. The rather strict fat-reduced diet given to the Trappist monks brought their LDL down much more than HDL. A less stringent diet in Oxford, given to people with blood fats high enough to have them referred to a hospital clinic, did the same. In a group of thirteen patients put on a fat-reduced diet containing margarine and cooking oil instead of butter and lard, their average cholesterols came down from about 300 to 260, while the proportion of HDL actually rose.

In the last few years a quite different potential has emerged for this type of low-fat diet. A research team in North Karelia, Finland, found that the diet not only reduced serum cholesterol by 13 per cent but also brought down blood pressure. A group of about thirty Finnish volunteers aged between thirty and fifty spent six weeks on a diet that provided only about half their usual fat intake and contained equal amounts of saturated and unsaturated fats. This was a great change from what they usually ate, but it was put together quite easily using skimmed milk, lean meat, low-fat sausage and low-fat cheese. At the end of the six weeks they went back to eating their normal meals. While they were on the diet their cholesterol levels fell and their blood pressures came down appreciably as well. The fall was seen in subjects with both normal and raised blood pressures. When they went back to their normal diets, pressures rose again.

The Finnish researchers suggest that '. . . change in dietary fats seems a promising method for the non-pharmacological [that is to say, drug-free] treatment and prevention of hypertension'. If so, the low-fat diet may have particular benefits, at least for those with a blood pressure problem.

8. Aerobics and Beta-blockade

According to the National Institutes of Health, sixty million Americans have high blood pressure. The proportion in Britain is probably similar. Physicians call it 'hypertension', which doesn't mean very much until we know what they call 'normal', and that's not as simple as you might think.

When your heart contracts, it pumps blood into your arteries. When it expands again it receives the blood which has been round your body back from your veins. So we all have two blood pressures, a higher one when the heart is emptying, and a lower one when it is filling again. Since a heart beat is known medically as a *systole*, the first pressure is called 'systolic'. I referred to it earlier as the 'pumping pressure'. Refilling is called *diastole*, so the second pressure is called 'diastolic'. Both of them are measured by putting an inflatable cuff around your arm and blowing it up until the cuff pressure outside the artery is equal to your blood pressure inside. It's a ritual performed at least a hundred million times every year in the USA alone. The cuff connects to a column of mercury, and so pressures are expressed as the weight of a mercury column so many centimetres high. Newer units have been introduced, but we can expect blood pressures to go on being recorded as, say, 140/90 (systolic/ diastolic) millimetres of mercury (written as mm Hg) for many years to come.

What then is a normal blood pressure? It's the average pressure you might expect to find in a group of apparently healthy people, bearing in mind that in Western countries systolic pressure increases about 3 mm for every five years that we get older. But the average for any group may be far from the ideal. Some specialists believe that an ideal pressure is the lowest you can have without fainting – say 100/60. They think so because as your pressure rises, the problems that go with it increase as well.

Some years ago an expert group commissioned by the World Health Organization decided that the highest blood pressure that could be called *normal* was 140/90. Pressures between that and 160/95 are called *borderline*, and if your blood pressure is more than 160/95 then, according to WHO, you have hypertension. On this basis, twenty-five million Americans are borderline, and another thirty-five million have their pressures definitely raised. And raised blood pressure increases your risk of suffering either from a stroke or from a coronary.

Strokes result from increased blood pressure in the arteries supplying the brain. The arterial wall bursts and blood seeps out into the brain itself. Alternatively, an artery may get blocked up with fragments of atheroma or blood clots, and the part of the brain that it supplies simply dies off – a brain infarction just like an infarction in the heart. Populations with low blood pressure have few strokes. Those where it is high have many. The Japanese, for example, are among the world leaders for both stroke and hypertension. For Britons and Americans too, your chances of a stroke are directly related to your blood pressure level.

The other result of hypertension is coronary disease. As the pressure in the artery rises, its walls are more likely to get damaged. Substances like cholesterol or platelets then get into the muscle layers and the result is atheroma. The Pooling Project compared the coronary risks for men with the highest blood pressures (systolic or diastolic) to those with the lowest. Both answers came out the same – for the high pressure group the risk was doubled.

But many of the men in the Pooling Project were only mild hypertensives and the Project didn't look at strokes at all. A better idea of the real dangers of hypertension comes from the now famous statistics produced by the Metropolitan Life Insurance Company. They compared life expectancies at various levels, considering deaths from all pressure-related causes. In the 1960s when the calculations were made, a thirty-five-year-old man with a blood pressure of 120/80 could expect to die at seventy-six. If his pressure was 140/95 then his departure was scheduled for sixty-seven, but if it was 150/100 then he was likely to die at sixty. Obviously the risk increases sharply when the pressure does. A level of 150/100 isn't spectacular if you consider the population as a whole. But it's enough to shorten your life by fifteen years.

It is remarkable that blood pressure measured on one single occasion, a so-called 'casual' reading, predicts future death or illness at all, because every doctor knows that casual readings can vary so much. If the patient had to rush across town; if he is having an insurance medical and is afraid of being rated; if the examination will influence his job prospects; or if he simply doesn't like doctors; all of these possibilities can put his pressure up. Knowing this, the doctor takes it several times and usually finds a fall from the first reading to the last, as his patient gets more familiar with the surroundings. Sometimes, a nurse will take it. Being less frightening than doctors, nurses often obtain lower readings. And when these same patients take their own pressures at home, they are often lower still.

But the ups and downs that we show in the doctor's office are nothing to what every one of us experiences during the course of an ordinary day. In the 1960s it became possible to measure blood pressure over the whole day in people going about their normal business. The highest pressures recorded during the twenty-four hours were more than double the lowest. One team of British cardiologists actually commented that if a systolic pressure of 150 means hypertension, then all of their patients were hypertensive at least some of the time.

But the twenty-four-hour studies also showed that our blood pressure stays a lot lower for much of the day. One group who followed it found that it starts to rise when we wake up and get involved in the daily routine – washing, dressing, getting the kids to school, getting ourselves to work. The peak occurs at mid-morning and from then on it falls slowly during the afternoon and evening to reach its lowest levels when we are asleep. At any time it can suddenly shoot up, as the result of a flash of anger, or of a shock, but for most of us the sudden rises fall again just as quickly. There are still arguments about what twenty-four-hour blood pressures are showing, but your average pressure over the day probably isn't very different from what you register in the doctor's surgery. So insurance companies were right to base their premiums on a single casual reading. Of course, they never doubted it – life insurance isn't a loss-making business.

Pleasure or pain, anger or excitement, can all produce short-term increases in blood pressure. Even talking can do it. But for most people they don't cause a sustained rise. What does? Amazingly enough, considering the time and money that are spent studying it, we're still not sure. Narrowing of the aorta will do it, and so will diseases of the kidneys and the arteries that supply them. Tumours of the adrenal glands can also produce sustained hypertension. But these complaints together make up no more than one in twenty (some experts would say no more than one in a hundred) of all cases of hypertension. For the others, the disease is said to be 'essential' – a medical term meaning that the cause is simply unknown. Often it results from several effects all acting together – physical and psychological too.

For example, hypertension may result from being overweight. Early results from Framingham made it look as though excessive overweight (obesity) was an important risk factor for coronary disease. Today, no one really thinks that it is, at least not unless your body weight is 20 per cent over the average, and the Pooling Project found being overweight to be the weakest of the coronary risks that it looked at. But obesity can certainly lead to hypertension, and bringing your weight down brings your blood pressure down too. Nor do you have to get all the way down to your ideal weight. If you are an obese hypertensive, even reducing your overweight burden by a third will show some benefit.

There has been a lot written about what your ideal weight should be. Remember, there was some doubt in Alameda County. Tables of 'desirable weight' for height were produced by the Metropolitan Life Insurance Company in the 1950s after they had recorded the deaths of more than four million people who had been through their examinations. More recently, some experts have questioned whether the Metropolitan figures are too low. For example, the records of employees at the Chicago People's Gas Company in 1975 showed the lowest death rates to occur in those men who were nearly a third heavier than the Metropolitan tables said they should have been. Other figures suggest that very thin people have an excessively high mortality. It seems that when the Duchess of Windsor said 'It's not possible to be too rich or too thin' she may have been only half right.

The latest analysis, a ten-year follow-up of over eight thousand men in Honolulu, leaves no doubt that the 20 per cent of those with the highest body weight (or rather 'body mass index', a ratio of height to weight) had more deaths from CHD than those who were leaner. The thinnest 40 per cent of men also had higher death rates – many from cancer.

But their higher death rate may not have been due to their body shape. As Nedra Belloc suggested, they were probably thin because they were already suffering from the effects of disease when they came to be weighed. In contrast, those who were lean all their lives – the ones with the lowest body mass index at age twenty-five – also had the lowest mortality in middle age. Meyer Friedman noticed the same thing many years ago. In 1969 he wrote: '. . . when we first see and examine a tall, quite thin, poorly muscled individual with flat forearms who is less than 55 years of age, we would be rather surprised if he were found to have clinical coronary artery disease.'

The most fashionable cause of hypertension is a high salt intake. The argument over salt and blood pressure is like the story that links dietary cholesterol with coronary disease. Communities who eat little salt have little hypertension. But those international comparisons are only true for large numbers. Like cholesterol, there seems to be no clear link between salt intake and blood pressure for you or me or any other single individual.

Some studies have been hopeful. A group of nineteen mild hypertensives in London with an average blood pressure of 156/98 were put on a salt-restricted diet and after only two weeks their pressures had come down by nearly 7 per cent. Two weeks back on salt and it went back up again. Now 7 per cent may not seem much, but a doctor who got this effect using drugs would be quite happy. And so a lot of physicians believe that salt restriction is always 'worth trying'. But it doesn't always work. When a group of eighteen hypertensives with an average pressure of 144/93 went through exactly the same salt restriction in a town in South Wales, it had no effect whatever. The low salt diet may work better for hypertensives with diastolic pressures nearer 100 than 90 – just the people whose doctors are likely to put them on drugs. So perhaps its future is in keeping down the total drug dose.

But to have any chance of working at all your salt intake has to be very much lower than it usually is. This means banning salt both from the kitchen and from the table. Even so, you will have to cook all your meals at home. A fried chicken take-away or a hamburger and french fries at a fast food joint both have more salt than the daily allowance for a low salt diet.

But where does the overdriver fit into this blood pressure story? If situations that we meet every day can cause sudden sharp rises in pressure, the natural question is whether, for him at least, having them repeated often enough can make the increase permanent.

Take just a few examples of the many that have been looked at. A British college lecturer in his early thirties went to his doctor with a diastolic pressure high enough to shorten his life appreciably. Instead of giving him drugs, the physician decided to follow him closely to see what happened. Over a period of six to seven years his blood pressure came back down to normal. The lecturer later admitted that at the time when it was raised he had felt 'a lot of tension'. In the same group of patients was a young, high-ranking architect employed by the county. He and his superior, the county clerk, did not always agree on policy. During a period of particular hostility the architect's blood pressure rose to 240/140, a high that today would call for instant treatment. But instead he too was closely watched and it came down again after the incident had been resolved.

Dr Peter Nixon, of the Charing Cross Hospital in London, described his results on over sixty hypertensives (blood pressures from 160/100 to 230/130) who came into hospital for examination. Part of his approach to treatment involves putting them to sleep, giving them light sedation and providing a warm and caring atmosphere. As a result, half of their pressures returned to normal, and only one in ten had no response at all.

Case histories like these show how anyone under pressure, Type A or B, may have to live with their problem for so long that without treatment their blood pressure might become permanently 're-set' at a higher level. We saw that a number of experts believe that this is exactly the way some borderline hypertensives get pushed over the edge. Others disagree. They can find no good evidence that disturbing your nervous system, even long term, will permanently alter your pressure.

But none of this may be basic to the overdriver's problem. He may not have re-set his blood pressure on any permanent basis. By raising it often enough in the course of the day; by exposing himself to enough spikes of arousal; by generating enough sudden volleys of sympathetic traffic, he can damage his health just as effectively, without ever appearing in the tables of Metropolitan Life. Overdrive means over-reaction, daily outbursts that a casual blood pressure reading in the doctor's office might miss altogether.

Even so, some overdrivers are hypertensive as well. And so the problem is not only to control their arousal surge, but to get their average blood pressures down too. Let's say you're one of them. Let's say that following your physician's advice you've reduced your weight, cut down the salt and much of the fat in your diet. But your blood pressure is still raised. What do you do then?

One thing you do is learn to relax. The next chapter will tell you how. But the other thing that either you do for yourself or that your doctor does for you, is to take your pressure regularly over a period of weeks before he even thinks about putting you on drugs. As well as visits to his surgery, it would be helpful if he lent you a pressure machine (or you bought one) to use yourself at home. Your pressure may well fall after a few weeks of simply measuring it. Even the county architect's frighteningly high levels came down again once the hassle had passed out of his life, and having their blood pressures recorded on a regular basis at home or in the clinic, has brought many hypertensives into the normal range. The World Health Organization, which largely reflects opinion within Europe and the Third World, now recommends that anyone with a diastolic pressure less than 100 mm Hg should have it followed for three months before any drugs are used. If in that time it comes down below 95 then they shouldn't be treated at all, so long as it stays there.

But in the United States, the philosophy is different. The first drug treatment to benefit hypertensives dates back to 1964. Strokes and heart failure were dramatically reduced in a group of men with diastolic pressures between 100 and 120 mm Hg – levels that today we would call 'severe'. In the later 1960s the Veterans Administration looked for benefits in treating lower pressures. They found them. There was a clear advantage in drug treatment for men with diastolics between 105 and 114. And today there can be few physicians anywhere in the world who doubt the wisdom of treating sustained diastolic pressures of 105 or more.

The VA study didn't produce any clear-cut benefits from treating men with diastolic pressures below 105. But one adult in every four in the Western world probably has a diastolic between 90 and 109. To throw light on this most important question, a trial with some four thousand volunteers was set up in Australia in 1973. Those with diastolics of 95 mm Hg or more were given drugs and their progress was followed for nearly four hours, at which point the organizers decided that they had the answer. They declared the benefits to be proved beyond doubt, and if the same treatment could have been applied to the whole Australian population they calculated that there would have been two thousand fewer strokes and seven thousand fewer episodes of cardiovascular disease each year.

However, on looking more closely at the Australian figures, it becomes clear that the benefit occurred in volunteers with pressures of 100 mm and beyond. Those running diastolics of 95 to 99 were to be carefully watched, but not treated. And over half the participants had a fall in blood pressure without getting any real treatment at all – either through knowing that they had been selected for attention or as the result of receiving dummy tablets.

What do physicians in the USA do with patients whose blood pressure, measured on several occasions, stubbornly stays between 95 and 100? They treat them. But then, they treat them for diastolic pressures of 90 mm as well. Most would claim to do so because of the results of the Hypertension Detection and Follow-up Program (HDFP), a five-year investigation costing $70 million, which involved screening more than a hundred and sixty thousand people in their homes. Nearly eleven thousand were located who had diastolic pressures of 90 mm Hg or more, and they were split into two groups. One received normal care and attention from their personal physician. The others got an intensive programme of anti-hypertensive therapy based on the HDFP clinic centres. They were given drugs, singly or in combination, to bring their pressures down. And I mean 'given'. Drugs, clinic visits, transport and laboratory costs were all free. Volunteers were actively encouraged to take their medication and in case of any problems, real or imaginary, a physician was on call day and night to deal with any queries. Waiting times were reduced to a minimum and appointments were made to suit the patients' convenience.

The results of this intensive programme were impressive. Over the five years that the study ran, the death rate came down by a fifth for patients receiving clinic attention whose diastolic pressures were 90 to 104 mm Hg when they were first recruited. The message seemed clear enough. As Dr Gerald Payne, the Project Officer for the HDFP, said at the Press Conference to launch the results in November 1979:

'Of the approximately 25 million Americans with so-called "mild" hypertension, millions are not being treated because they or their doctors feel there is little benefit in treating hypertension if it is in the mild range. Until now there wasn't clear scientific proof of the benefits of treating this group of patients.

'This study clearly demonstrates that the systematic, effective treatment of mild hypertension may reduce premature deaths by 20 per cent.

'*To the millions of Americans who have high blood pressure this study says:* get on treatment and *stay* on treatment. It will mean a much longer life . . . more years to spend with your loved ones.'

And who am I to argue? Except perhaps to point out that the HDFP isn't the usual way that Americans get their medical care. Free drugs, free doctors' time, free transport to the clinic, minimal waiting time and a special physician whose job is to answer the phone to you in the middle of the night are hardly normal.

In short, many European doctors believe that the HDFP wasn't so much a trial of anti-hypertensive drugs as a trial of the health-care system. If that level of care were available for everyone, there might not be a blood pressure problem. Also disturbing is the fact that in the mid-1970s, long before the HDFP reported its results, three-quarters of the doctors in New York State were said to be already treating diastolic pressures in the range 90–100 mm. The HDFP results didn't so much point to a course of action as confirm one that had already been going on for years.

Obviously, nothing I say is going to change any of this. But why, you might ask, should we be concerned about it? If taking drugs for your blood pressure were a short-term treatment with no drawbacks then the question of what level to start might not be so important. The problem is that once you go on to anti-hypertensives you can expect to be on them for the rest of your life. If you come off, then your pressure will probably climb back again. No one likes taking pills every day and many patients stop after a few weeks or months. Unless your pressure is very high you don't even know about it, because there are no headaches, palpitations or feelings of 'tension'. That's the whole problem about finding those people who do need treating – they have no symptoms to send them to their doctors. On the other hand, the effects of the pills may be all too obvious, and many hypertensives decide for themselves that they would rather feel well now and risk the consequences than go around feeling awful in the hope of some long-term benefit.

To understand the side-effects we need to know how the drugs work. There are three ways of getting your blood pressure down. The first is by reducing the total amount of fluid in your blood vessels. This is done by increasing urine flow, and the drugs that make you excrete more fluid more often are known as 'diuretics'. Secondly, your blood pressure may be due to contraction of the vessels that carry it. A second group of drugs, the 'vasodilators', make your blood vessels relax. A large bore pipe has less resistance than a narrow one. Thirdly, your raised pressure may be due to your heart beating too fast or too hard, forcing more fluid into the vessels than they can comfortably handle. To stop it working so hard we have the beta-blockers. You will remember that they block the catecholamine receptors on the heart's surface. This lessens the muscle's response, rather like putting a wedge under your accelerator to stop it going down to the floor.

You might think that these three treatments are quite separate and all the physician has to do is find out what is causing *yours* and give you the appropriate pill. But it doesn't happen that way. Although many young hypertensives have an increased cardiac output while many older ones develop narrowed arteries, most doctors can't say from a surgery examination whether your raised pressure is due to excess fluid, contracted vessels or an overactive heart. In practice, what many do is to put you on a particular drug and see if it works. If not, they include a second, and if that doesn't do it they add a third.

Eight out of ten patients manage to control their blood pressure with this 'triple therapy', but they do so at a cost. Drs Peter Stirling and Joe Eyer of the University of Pennsylvania have pointed out that the one organ that decides how high your blood pressure *should* be is your brain. Only your brain knows how much challenge there is in your environment, and how high your blood pressure has to be to meet it. If you bring the pressure down by altering one system, say the total amount of fluid in your body, then your brain may try to find other ways to push it up again. That may be why some patients need triple therapy, to overcome all the brain's efforts to keep your pressure up. Far better, Stirling and Eyer suggest, to reduce the arousal in your life. If you can do that, and your hypertension has not gone on for so long that it has become fixed, then your brain has a chance of bringing your blood pressure down to a level that matches your surroundings.

What are the side-effects that you might expect from anti-hypertensive drugs? Most of them can cause fatigue and weakness, sedation and depression and a falling off in sexual performance. Since diuretics reduce the blood volume they may disturb the balance of water and salts in your blood, which can lead to lethargy and weakness. A fall in potassium can produce arrhythmias. Though some diuretics are less of a problem than others, a surprisingly large number of patients with levels of potassium low enough to cause ventricular fibrillation were found to be taking diuretics for their hypertension. Some specialists even suggest that the reason why few, if any, trials of anti-hypertensives have shown a fall in the infarction rate (rather than a fall in strokes or total mortality) is because any beneficial effect was offset by an increase in fibrillation or sudden death. Almost as disturbing is the recent finding from a large-scale British anti-hypertensive trial that both gout and impotence were frequent enough among men on diuretics to be major reasons for their withdrawing from the study.

Vasodilators have their problems too. Some of them cause serious sedation. Others, because they reduce the resistance to blood flow, may lead to a sudden increase in pulse rate and cardiac output. If the heart is struggling already, this can cause angina, as the work rate of the myocardium gets ahead of its oxygen supply.

Then we have the beta-blockers, which have been quite rightly described as a real breakthrough in the treatment of angina and arrhythmias as well as hypertension. Their success in treating the first two depends on them slowing down the rate and force of the heart's contraction. Of course by doing so they reduce the maximum amount of work that it can do. In other words, you tire more easily, and you eventually have to resign yourself to not being able to do many of the things you could do before. As one physician – himself put on beta-blockade – told Stirling and Eyer: 'When I take them, I can't walk up a hill.' So he didn't take them.

Beta-blockers are targeted on receptors in the myocardium. But other receptors in many other parts of the body can get blocked as well, with results that could be serious if they weren't watched for. For example, the airways in the lungs expand under the influence of catecholamines. In someone on beta-blockers they can't do so, and the result is that asthmatics can't use them at all. Even people with breathing problems so mild that they didn't regard themselves as asthmatics have had frightening experiences and most doctors today will examine your airways before they put you on these drugs. There are beta-receptors on blood vessels too, and blocking these may reduce the circulation, say in your legs. Specialists have even associated their use with coronary spasms – passing angina with no permanent coronary blockage. Some of these problems are lessened by using drugs specially tailored to be 'selective' for the myocardium. But even selective beta-blockers may have a spill-over.

Then there are the more 'subjective' side-effects – vivid nightmares, depression and dizziness, all reported by patients on beta-blockade. Finally there are the ill effects that you don't know anything about. Some beta-blockers reduce HDL and increase LDL – the reverse of what you apparently need to avoid atheroma. But even diuretics can cause HDL to fall and total cholesterol to rise.

No one it seems, knowing all this, would choose to go on to beta-blockers if there were effective non-drug possibilities open to them. Or would they? The one group who might are the ones you would least expect. Some of the most frantic hard-core Type As might just see a pill as their salvation.

The overdriver seems to be addicted to noradrenaline. He behaves in many ways like a rat that keeps on stimulating its own brain centres and ignores pain, hunger or fatigue. And so a number of people interested in Type A (including Malcolm Carruthers, Ray Rosenman and even myself) have wondered if one could 'disconnect' the stimulation that the overdriver does it all for from the physical damage that his behaviour causes to his body.

For the extreme A1 there may be little hope of changing his behaviour or his attitude in the Type B direction. So what we might try to do is reduce the effects that his self-destructive way of life has on his heart. Such a hard case simply won't be interested in wasting his precious time with a counsellor, or in a group, trying to gain insight into his behaviour. He's just too busy, too hostile or both. But might he be persuaded to take a pill? If he has hypertension, even worse if he has angina, then he will be used to medication already. An extra tablet might just be tolerable.

The pills would be beta-blockers of course. They would let his catecholamine jags go on without interruption – the highs he couldn't do without. But by blocking many of his beta-receptors, his heart rate and perhaps his blood pressure too might stay within reasonable bounds. He might not keep on pouring out free fatty acids, with the risk of arrhythmias that they produce, and his coronary arteries might not keep narrowing.

Unfortunately, we don't really know what beta-blockers actually do to Type As. The closest look at the question so far comes from the Walter Reed Army Medical Center in Maryland. Dr David Krantz and his colleagues at the Uniformed Services University School of Medicine were impressed by a small-scale comparison made in Bonn, West Germany, between Type A patients receiving a beta-blocker and those on a diuretic. Their Type A intensity (as measured by the structured interview) fell during their time on beta-blockade. But there was no similar effect from the diuretic. It seemed that reducing the activity of the sympathetic nervous system also reduced their Type A behaviour. And to Krantz and his colleagues that made good sense.

They had already looked at what happens to Type As when they undergo coronary by-pass surgery, following an earlier finding that even under deep general anaesthesia, Type As showed more sympathetic reactivity than Type Bs. They did structured interviews on a group of twenty-seven men, mostly in their early fifties, coming to have their coronary arteries by-passed with a vein graft. There were two Type A1s and nineteen Type A2s in the group – itself an indication of how Type As predominate among individuals at high risk of coronary attack.

The men's blood pressures were recorded throughout the surgery and the highest systolic responses – even when they were under full anaesthesia an hour into the operation – were shown by the Type As. This suggested that Type A itself might be partly '. . . an excessive sympathetic response to environmental stressors', a response that occurred even when the sufferer was too deeply anaesthetized to know anything about it.

At first glance this seems to turn the usual view of the Type A on its head. Most specialists have always said that his behaviour results from his conscious interaction with his surroundings, and more especially with the people in them. It's the demands of the moment that produce that sinking, time-urgent feeling and it is the burden of other people slowing you down that leads to anger. Now here comes the suggestion that Type A has its roots so far below the surface as to be unconscious. Can both ideas be right?

Yes they can. What the Maryland team are suggesting is that early in his life the Type A's sympathetic system goes through so many cycles of conscious arousal that the reaction becomes programmed in. The automatic pilot takes over, so that in later life not only does he react to the hassles that he is conscious of, but his sympathetic system is conditioned to react without him even knowing about it. Such reactions may be responsible *both* for the appearance of the behaviour and for whatever it is that links the behaviour to the disease.

But back to beta-blockers. Of the eighty or more patients who had structured interviews at the Walter Reed, sixty-five were already being given a beta-blocker called *propranolol*. The research team had an opportunity to compare them with the twenty-three who weren't. The propranolol-treated patients had lower total Type A scores. A number of their speech characteristics, such as loud and explosive, and rapid and accelerated, were reduced, as was their potential for hostility. The heart rate reactions of patients during the structured interview were also lessened as the result of beta-blockade, but not as the result of taking diuretics.

We shouldn't read too much into these results. They relate to patients taking their medication as Krantz found them, and they don't add up to a before-and-after drug trial. Nor do they answer the question of *why* beta-blockade should bring Type A levels down. But the Walter Reed group offer an intriguing explanation.

When our sympathetic system starts to take over, we know about it. Our heart starts to pound and our hands may start to shake. We feel generally disturbed. Just realizing that can make it worse. With anxious people, their inner anxieties increase as they notice these things happening: 'I'm getting anxious again. Look, I can feel it.' They get into a vicious circle and some doctors prescribe low doses of beta-blockers to calm their sympathetic system and reduce their anxiety – from the outside in.

Now Type As are not particularly anxious, but a similar reaction might take over. Say an A1 starts to interact with someone else. As a result, his heart rate and blood pressure go up. As he becomes aware of his responses, they reinforce his behaviour. His tempo quickens and his voice style becomes more energetic. He too gets caught in a cycle of positive feedback, like a microphone feeding into a loudspeaker. If he is put on beta-blockers he is still likely to get energized by the presence of other people, but his sympathetic response is reduced. His catecholamines can't plug into all of their receptors and if he doesn't become aware of so many reactions, the feedback doesn't start to amplify. In short, his sympathetic system doesn't spiral out of control.

So the theory holds together. But are we really likely to see beta-blockers as a practical treatment of Type A? Personally, I don't think so. Nor do I think we should, except perhaps for the most self-destructive. As Krantz's group themselves point out, we don't yet know whether these drugs will actually reduce the risk of coronary disease that results from being Type A. You might expect them to. Propranolol prevents your heart rate taking off when you're in a difficult situation. But blood pressure responses didn't fall in Krantz's study and physicians in Austria have found that rises in diastolic pressures during mental arithmetic were actually higher when healthy young volunteers were taking propranolol than when they were taking no drugs at all. There are other worries as well. A group of healthy young men in London taking beta-blockers as part of an experiment, were asked to exercise on a bicycle. Blood samples were taken for adrenaline and noradrenaline and their catecholamine responses to exercise were actually found to be *higher* on some beta-blockers than when they were taking no medication at all.

So apart from fatigue and 'exercise intolerance' there may be other drug-related effects that can hardly be beneficial either. Add to that the fact that beta-blockade might encourage you to put yourself in situations that over-stimulate your sympathetic system without you even knowing it, and the fact that '. . . some patients already reject medication with beta-blockers because of the reduced capacity for emotional reactions which they produce' and they don't seem to hold a lot of promise in this direction.

Type As who have had an infarction will almost certainly be getting beta-blockade already – like many of the patients that Krantz interviewed. But it has nothing to do with their behaviour. They get the drugs to protect their hearts against a second infarction. And while beta-blockers might also be valuable for some non-infarcted patients with other symptoms, their use in 'healthy' people (even Type A1s if they don't have hypertension or angina) seems doubtful. Physicians use drugs to treat symptoms not to stop symptoms from occurring, particularly if there are non-drug alternatives.

And in this case there are. Exercise is one of them.

Take the experience of some two hundred sedentary middle-aged men who joined the Epic Health Club Inc. in Montreal and went through a six-month conditioning programme. For a two-hourly session every week they jogged, did light gymnastics (callisthenics) and played volleyball. They were also encouraged to do ten to fifteen minutes of callisthenics every day at home. Before they started they had a medical check-up which showed that about forty of them were borderline hypertensives, with systolics of 140–159 mm Hg and diastolics of 90–95. The rest, with pressures less than 140/90, were normotensive. At the end of the six-month programme their blood pressures were measured again. Both groups showed a fall and for the hypertensives it was quite striking – 15 mm systolic and 8 mm diastolic – as good as you might expect with a drug.

Exercise may be useful for people who are on drugs already, to help keep their dosage down, but still keep their pressures normal. Drs John L. Boyer and Fred W. Kasch at San Diego State College enrolled twenty-three middle-aged men who had been hypertensive (diastolics over 105) for at least a year, and who were all on medication, into a six-month programme of interval training where short bursts of activity are separated by periods of rest. The group met for two days every week. How hard they were training was judged from their pulse rate. The aim was to have the men working at three-quarters of their maximum heart rate (say 145 beats per minute for a man of forty-five) and to have them take their own pulse during the session so that they could keep inside their own limits. After six months the hypertensives' pressures were down by an average of about 12 mm (both systolic and diastolic) – a very worthwhile reduction.

The drugs the men had continued to take all this time were mainly diuretics and vasodilators. None of them were on beta-blockers and if they had been the results might have been different. We have seen that exercise and beta-blockers simply don't go together. Beta-blockade so reduces exercise performance that many runners who are put on them confess to taking themselves off again before an event.

What does exercise do apart from bringing raised blood pressure down? What most people do it for is to reduce their weight, and physical activity will certainly cause weight reduction. But it's a slow process, unless you live in a cold climate. At the University of Toronto, six obese volunteers lost an average of 10 lbs in ten days as a result of three and a half hours of vigorous daily exercise. But they were working out in a special cold chamber at −34°C (about −29°F). In warmer climates and with more moderate exercise, the losses are smaller. One estimate put the weight lost as a result of half an hour's daily walking at only 1½ lbs per month, although if you scale this up it becomes 180 lbs (a fair-sized man's body weight) every ten years.

And what about cholesterol – does that go down with physical activity? Not by very much, perhaps 10 per cent. But more important than total cholesterol is the proportion of HDL. Populations with high levels of HDL seem to have low coronary rates, and certainly HDL is high in well-trained athletes. The Stanford Heart Disease Prevention Program is a multi-media campaign to encourage the populations of particular towns in California to take up a variety of health practices, exercise among them. At an early stage of the programme they decided to look at the effects of exercise in a group of men, many of whom had at one time been physically unfit, overweight smokers, but who had then taken up running and had been running for seven years. A group of forty-one of them (average age forty-seven) was compared with a similar group who took no exercise at all. There wasn't much difference in their total cholesterols (200 mg/100 ml in the runners; 210 in the controls) but the runners' LDL fractions (cholesterol being carried to the arteries) were 10 per cent lower and their HDLs (cholesterol being carried out of the arteries) were 30 per cent higher than in the sedentary men. The blood fats in these runners were like those in young women, who of course have the lowest coronary rates of all.

Unfortunately the exercise story has its negative side, and anyone who thought that running was going to solve all their health problems will have to think again. Some quite careful investigations have failed to show even the slightest benefit from an exercise programme. A research team at the Adelaide College of Art and Education in Australia enrolled about four hundred sedentary men of all ages from twenty to sixty-five into a three-month training schedule made up of twice-weekly sessions of callisthenics, running and volleyball. Before they joined they had their major risk factors measured (and pretty frightening they were too, in this 'typical' Australian population, with one in five showing a diastolic pressure over 95 and one in three having a serum total cholesterol over 250). At the end of the course they were encouraged to carry on exercising at home and five years later those of them who could be traced had their risk factors measured again. They were no different. Smoking, blood pressure and cholesterol were the same as they had been before the programme started. Perhaps this meant that most of them had given up exercising as soon as the course was over. And many of them had. But even among the one in three who had persisted with two hours of moderate to heavy exercise every week, their risk factors didn't change.

Exercise buffs will say that two hours a week simply wasn't a fair test. But it was enough to make their hearts fitter, which clearly isn't the same thing. Your heart rate, both during exercise and when you're at rest, falls quite noticeably as the result of regular work-outs. While an untrained person may have a pulse rate of 70–80 beats per minute, a well-trained athlete may have a rate of only 30. Add the fact that heavy training may produce a very abnormal-looking (though apparently healthy) electrocardiogram and some cardiologists think that athletes should wear a tag round their neck, like haemophiliacs or diabetics, to say that they are runners. That way, if they have a street accident, the physicians at the hospital won't automatically assume they've had a coronary.

Exercise also increases the amount of work that your heart can do. It reduces the effort that your myocardium has to make to pump blood round your body, either at rest or when your muscles are working hard. So 'cardiovascular fitness' means your heart being able to cope more effectively with the demands that are placed on it every day.

What it doesn't mean is a reduced risk of your having a heart attack. There have been many attempts to prove that exercise prevents coronaries, and many claims that it has been proved, but, like the diet and cholesterol studies, none of them stand up to scrutiny.

I hesitate to say this at a time when there are millions of runners in Britain and the United States. All of them (all of us) want to hear that running lengthens your life. But we simply can't be sure that it does. We saw the findings from Alameda County, and there have been even more impressive studies than that, like the observation of six thousand Californian longshoremen, comparing the death rates of those with heavy and those with lighter jobs, and the even larger follow-up of seventeen thousand Harvard alumni to see whether taking part in college athletics had any influence on their life span. Both of these studies, which were led by Dr Ralph S. Paffenbarger Jr, of the California State Department of Public Health, deserve our respect for their sheer size and organization. Both suggest that physical activity, either on the job or during leisure, prolongs life.

But neither of them prove it. The problem is the same that we found in Alameda County – self-selection. The longshoremen with the heavier work and the Harvard athletes may have been healthier to begin with. This head start might have made them better on the job or more effective on the team. And it might have also made them tougher – less prone to disease or death. The physical effort they had to make may have been almost incidental and Paffenbarger himself has admitted as much when discussing the fall in American death rates: 'Neither the trends of increasing energy expenditure since the late 1960s nor the proportion of Americans now involved in high levels of energy output, would seem to represent major factors in the CHD decline observed over the last decade.'

Of course, all this talk about 'may' and 'might have' won't stop the enthusiasts from believing that their work-outs are adding years to their lives. What they ought to settle for is that exercise is adding life to their years. The improvement in vigour, self-image and well-being that many exercisers experience is now so well known that it has become a subject of study in itself. Some of the same investigators in North Carolina who looked at hostility and death rates have also turned their attention to the effects of aerobics. They found that after ten weeks of walking and jogging, volunteers were less anxious, tense, tired and depressed than a similar group who didn't go through the same routine.

The effect on depression is particularly interesting. A research team in the Department of Psychiatry at the

University of Wisconsin found that for the treatment of moderate depression, a ten-week exercise programme seemed to be as effective as psychotherapy. And it costs far less. The way it works isn't clear, but the sense of mastering your environment that comes with being able to run must have something to do with it. So too must the simple distraction. It is really quite difficult to run and carry on thinking about your depression at the same time. And it's even possible that exercise changes your brain biochemistry in the way that some antidepressant drugs are thought to do.

So exercise has real benefits. But it has real risks as well, and it would be foolish, perhaps even fatal, to ignore them – a message that applies to the overdriver more than to anyone else.

There is no longer any doubt that exercise kills people. Not many people perhaps, compared to the number who are exercising. And there are precautions you can take to lessen the chance of it killing you. But the possibility of a fatal heart attack is something that every runner should consider before he takes it up.

Some specialists play the risks down. One well-known study of six thousand people who collapsed during exercise or work concluded that 'no case was encountered of a previously healthy individual having died suddenly from excessive exertion'. But how many of us have a coronary system that you could call healthy? Even young soldiers in Korea had a surprising amount of atheroma. And when sudden deaths in an earlier generation of soldiers were examined, just after World War II, they were clearly associated with vigorous exercise. These young men spent a third of their time asleep, but only one fatal seizure in·seven occurred while they slept. By contrast, they spent only half as much time in strenuous activity, but the attack rate during exercise was twice as high.

Meyer Friedman, together with Ray Rosenman and others, examined this question in a much-quoted study of fifty-nine men who died suddenly or instantaneously in California. Of the instantaneous deaths, at least a third had been involved in strenuous exertion immediately beforehand. Most of them had narrowed coronary arteries. The cause of death was generally fibrillation, as the coronary blood supply was not able to keep pace with the heart's sudden exertional demand for oxygen.

Friedman is well known (if not well regarded) among American cardiologists for condemning exercise out of hand. Since there were some two hundred thousand instantaneous deaths annually in the United States in the mid-1970s, he estimated that a third of them (say sixty thousand) might have been due to exertion. As early as 1975 he wrote to me saying that '. . . as *clinicians* we are getting sick and tired of having both patients and friends dying after jogging, tennis, shovelling snow, etc. And what evidence is there that heart-rate-increasing exercise rids an artery of its fibrous calcified plaques? What good is a finely trained neuromuscular unit if its fuel lines close up?'

Most other physicians have a different opinion. Even so, there is no denying the figures. Tens of thousands of exercise tests have been done in cardiology centres to look for evidence of coronary disease. Professor Roy J. Shephard of the School of Physical Health and Education in Toronto, who has as much experience of exercise testing as anyone, calculates that such procedures increase the risk of an immediate coronary attack by at least four times. When groups are exercising together, the risks are greater, because inevitably some individuals try to out-perform the others. In Shephard's view this is not necessarily a reason to abandon exercise testing. The test is done under full medical supervision with a defibrillator handy, and if you're going to have a coronary there could be no better time to do so. But

I doubt if many patients are convinced.

Because of the risks of taking up exercise, especially if you are over thirty-five, all the fitness guides tell you to go and have a check-up with your doctor first. If he clears you then you're OK. But unfortunately you're not. Your doctor can look for the signs that say you definitely shouldn't exercise (angina, uncontrolled high blood pressure, excessive weight and so on) but he can't definitely pass you as fit. You may have coronary atheroma that simply doesn't show.

When your physician (or your favourite jogging manual, which is quite probably written by a physician) tells you to get yourself an exercise test before you start, he is suggesting that you invest in what Shephard calls 'defensive medicine'. The test doesn't so much cover you from the danger of an attack as cover the doctor from the danger of being sued by your next of kin. Even the Cardiology Branch of the National Heart, Lung and Blood Institute has concluded that the exercise electrocardiogram taken while you climb up and down on a pair of steps or walk on a treadmill is of 'very limited value' in diagnosing coronary artery disease in any individual patient. Attempts are being made to improve it, but as Friedman again commented in 1975, 'we would not allow men over thirty-five years of age to exercise violently even if their treadmill ECGs appeared normal'.

So the key to deriving benefit (and pleasure) from your exercise programme is to pursue it in a non-violent way. Overdrivers may find that difficult, but the message is more important for them than for anyone else.

How much exercise do you need to get fit and keep fit? Certainly not thirty-nine miles a week, like the runners in the Stanford Project. Most specialists agree that you can get fit with three or four sessions a week each lasting for an hour. Once you've got your pulse down and made your heart more efficient you can keep it that way with rather less – perhaps as little as three weekly sessions, each of half an hour.

The key question is how hard you need to train. The best training effect on your heart appears when you work hard enough to have to breathe at three-quarters of your maximum oxygen intake. But on its own that advice is about as useful as saying reduce your saturated fat to 10 per cent of total calories. Like diet, we need practical advice about how to do it.

One guide is your pulse rate. Oxygen intake and heart rate are linked, so you can use your pulse to tell you how hard you are working. But your highest pulse rate depends on your age, and there is no simple formula that you can work out for yourself. You have to have it worked out for you, either by your physician or (more likely) you can get it from a book or an exercise record. I already mentioned the San Diego target pulse rate of 145 for a forty-five-year-old man – a rate to work up to and one to stay inside. But taking your own pulse during or immediately after exercise is not easy, and people tend to over-estimate how fit they are if they rely on their heart rate. A simpler rule has been suggested by Professor Peter Fentem of the University Hospital in Nottingham. It's really very simple – don't exercise beyond the point where you can comfortably talk to someone exercising with you.

Experienced runners will object that this is too conservative. It falls some way below the oxygen intake that gives the greatest training effect. Maybe it does, but it's quite hard enough to make you, and keep you, adequately fit, and if it stops you from pushing yourself into the danger zone it may also save your life. While we're on the subject, there are a few other things that you should never do. Never carry on exercising if you notice even the slightest pain in your chest; if you start to feel dizzy or light-headed, or if you start to be overcome by fatigue. And at all costs avoid competition. If you are Type A, try to take up Type B running. It doesn't matter if you're not the fastest in your group, or if today's time is slower than yesterday's – who's counting, except you?

And if that seems like advice for pansies, look at what happens to real men when they go after their sport until it hurts. Professor L. H. Opie of the Groot Schuur Hospital in Cape Town, famous as the site of the world's first heart transplant, collected together information on twenty-one South African sportsmen who met sudden or unexpected deaths. Eighteen of them were found to have coronary artery disease. Either they didn't know it or they simply ignored the signs.

For example, a yachtsman who had a suspected heart attack ten years previously rejected all advice to stay on land and died after a race in bad weather. A runner who had suffered a heart attack some years before insisted on 'fighting it' by running seven miles a day. He died while doing do. A tennis club champion dropped dead after defending his title against a younger opponent, and a middle-aged referee with angina and a positive ECG exercise tests, who insisted on finishing the match despite the pain in his chest, died under the shower.

The New York Marathon also has its share of self-inflicted injuries. In the 1978 event, a forty-nine-year-old runner started to feel chest pains when he was four miles into the race. He insisted on pushing himself for another four miles before he collapsed with an infarction. A second enthusiast of the same age never actually made the big event. Two months before the race he had fallen unconscious at the end of a hard run. He ignored it and went on training. A month later he died after another training session. He had a T-shirt that said 'You haven't really run a good marathon until you drop dead at the finish line'. It seems that he succeeded.

Now a hundred thousand marathoners are going to tell me that deaths like these are the exception. And of course they are. But if it happens to you, your dependants may take a different view. Exercise addiction and the tolerance to pain that it produces are mixed blessings. The easiest way to minimize the risk is to follow a well-tried system, like Dr Kenneth H. Cooper's *Aerobics* or the later *New Aerobics* that suggest a tailor-made programme for your particular fitness level, starting modestly with walking exercises and working your way up slowly. All the Type A has to do is to follow the programme and restrain his wish to start in the middle.

Apart from the cardiovascular benefits that anyone, overdriver or not, can derive from a sensible programme, it seems that Type As can get a special bonus. In a nine-month exercise routine in California, running more than three and a half miles a week '. . . conferred a high probability of reducing Type A behavior. Among runners many changed by one entire category.' And running, it seems, prevented sedentary men from increasing their Type A scores. In North Carolina, Type As undertaking a ten-week programme (three miles of jogging three times a week) showed a fall in blood pressure and body weight, and a rise in HDL. And in addition, their JAS Type A scores fell by a third. So exercise gives a special benefit to Type As, as long as they go about it with a Type B approach.

Of course, changing *any* coronary risk probably benefits the Type A more than anyone else. He has an extra, doubling risk factor that Bs and Xs don't share, and that multiplies his coronary load. So we have to look for ways of changing that as well. We have to find sensible answers for the overdriver who tells us that he's got his 'conventional' risk factors under control but who still has a question: 'My diet's OK,' he says, 'I'm normotensive, I've kicked cigarettes and I run for pleasure. But when the pressure's on my reactions still shoot right off the chart. So what else can I do to help myself?'

9. Relaxing is a Skill

Thirty years ago a team of physicians at New York's Belle Vue Hospital developed an electronic gun for treating hypertension. A coil of wire two feet high was connected to a 15,000 volt electrical supply. Long blue sparks shot out of the top when the power was switched on. Wired up to the coil was a tubular gun barrel, the end of which glowed white hot. The whole thing was connected to a TV screen that displayed a series of wavy lines, representing the discharge of electronic rays. Patients sat in front of the gun in a darkened room. They were told that it had been very successful in treating high blood pressure in the past. It was then aimed at their chest and turned on for anything between one and five minutes.

It worked. In the 1950s, drug therapy for hypertension was still new. Many hypertensives were walking around with very high pressures indeed, and the patients in this study had levels up to 215/138. But more than half of those treated with the gun had systolic falls of more than 35 mm Hg and drops in diastolic greater than 25 mm Hg.

Of course, the whole thing was a charade. The gun didn't generate rays at all. Its tip was made 'white hot' by a light bulb inside, and the high voltage coil with its glowing discharge (like something out of Boris Karloff's laboratory) was just for show. What it actually did, this gun that the research team admitted was 'not recommended for clinical application', was dramatically to reinforce the reassurance and medical care that the hypertensive patients were getting from the doctors. Many of them believed that the whole treatment package was going to do them good, and for a lot of them it did.

Nothing has changed. If we bring the clock forward a quarter century, we can see just the same effects in an updated form. No one believes in ray guns and 1950s sci-fi any more, but Professor W. Stuart Agras and his associates at Stanford University Medical Center did something similar in the early 1980s with the effects of muscle relaxation on blood pressure. They recruited thirty hypertensives using a newspaper advertisement, and took them into hospital for a day. They were taught a type of muscle relaxation that we will look at shortly. They learned how to tense and relax their muscles in sequence, at the same time paying attention to the different feelings of being tight and being relaxed. They went through three of these relaxation sessions on the same day. Each one lasted for about twenty minutes and blood pressures were measured before and after each.

When they arrived at the hospital, before they learned the method, the patients were briefed about what it was and how it worked. Half of them were told that its effect would be immediate. The others were given a different story – that relaxation works, but its effects might be delayed. Indeed, they might even see a rise in pressure before it started to go down again.

They were all taught exactly the same relaxation routine, but their response depended on what they'd been told. Those who believed in an immediate effect experienced one. Their systolic pressures went down by 17 mm Hg from the first session to the last. But those who had been told to expect a delay showed a drop of less than 3 mm. It all depended on the instructions.

Both the ray gun and the relaxation training show how very sensitive your blood pressure is to your mental state. So far we have seen hassle or distress pushing it up, but reassurance and relaxation can bring it down again. With relaxation, you've got to believe it's going to work. At least, you've got to give it a fair try. Healthy scepticism is OK, but if you deliberately set out to prove it's garbage, then you'll succeed – in your own case at least. And that's one reason why some psychologists doubt whether you can really learn it from a book, or a record. They believe that you're better off learning it from a therapist, either individually or in a group. He can tell you what and how you're doing, and actually show you your blood pressure coming down. The fall isn't generally as great as you can get with drugs, but most of us don't need a fall that large. What Stuart Agras confirmed was that relaxation doesn't have an automatic effect, like a beta-blocker might. As we've seen so often, the world you live in and the way you respond to that world will affect the results.

Most of us aren't hypertensives. Even the majority of Type As and hot responders have normal blood pressures *most of the time*. So why is it worth our while bothering with relaxation or biofeedback or meditation or any of the other non-drug methods for getting blood pressure down? The answer is that *most of the time* isn't good enough. The overdriver sends his pressure up perhaps twenty times a day. Sure, it may come down again, but the damage has been done. What he needs is some simple technique to practise the moment he starts to feel it rise. Then he might be able to stop it shooting off the chart. And that's exactly where most of the research is being concentrated at present – on teaching you and me how to keep our blood pressure low most of the time, how to recognize when it's just about to take off and, most importantly, how to switch the control on when you need it.

Let's start with relaxation. As well as a treatment for hypertensives, it is also the basis for many other types of self-management. Until you've developed some ability to relax, you can't gain much insight into your problem. So anyone looking to control their Type A or bring their hot responses into line, really can't avoid some form of relaxation training. But that doesn't simply mean the ability to sit quietly or 'take it easy'. Real relaxation is much more than that. Most of us are more tense than we realize, most of the time. Getting rid of that tension is a skill, like driving a car, and in the same way it has to be actively learned until, like driving, it becomes automatic. Once you do, it goes so much further than simply 'taking it easy', that experiments on relaxation often use people just sitting reading or watching TV as a relatively tense comparison group.

There are many forms of relaxation training, but most of them owe something to Dr Edmund Jacobson, a physiologist who worked at Harvard between the two World Wars. In the 1920s and 1930s Jacobson published his procedure for *progressive muscle relaxation*, and continued working on it in Chicago well into the 1960s. Progressive relaxation involves the tensing and relaxing of sixteen separate muscle groups. In Jacobson's original work, learning to relax a single group might take five to ten hourly sessions, and so a total of fifty or more training periods was not at all unusual – far more than most of us would even contemplate today.

Jacobson himself found that his relaxation procedure reduced both pulse rate and blood pressure. But such a long-term, complicated business might never have become popular if it hadn't also been applied to something quite different. In the late 1940s Dr Joseph Wolpe, one of the pioneers of behaviour therapy, was looking for ways of treating anxiety, particularly the habitual fears or phobias that some people have, for example of snakes, spiders, or small or large spaces. His method involved exposing the sufferers first in imagination then in reality to the things that they feared, but very gradually, over many visits. For example, during the first session the snake might be in a cage on the other side of the room. Many weeks went by before the phobic patients progressively learned to cross the room, open the cage and eventually handle the snake. To make this 'desensitization' more painless, the phobic was taught to relax, in the belief that relaxation reduced the fear and allowed the patient to approach the frightening object more quickly. Today there is some disagreement among the experts about whether Wolpe was right, and whether relaxation really does make desensitization easier. But either way, Jacobson-based relaxation is now part of the psychotherapist's tool-kit.

To show how it works I'll quote an example from a well-known relaxation training manual written for therapists in 1973 by Drs Douglas A. Bernstein and Thomas D. Borkovec, then at the University of Iowa. It represents a typical introductory session, with the therapist explaining to a new client what it is that he will be doing.

. . . The purpose of this first session is to help you learn to become deeply relaxed, perhaps more relaxed than you've ever been before, and we can begin this session by going over the muscle groups that we're going to be dealing with in relaxation training. At this point in training, there are sixteen muscle groups to be dealt with, sixteen groups which are tensed and relaxed. As your skill develops, this number will be reduced significantly.

We will begin training with the hand and forearm . . . I'll ask you to tense the muscles in the right hand and right lower arm by making a tight fist. Now you should be able to feel tension in the hand, over the knuckles, and up into the lower arm. Can you feel that tension? O.K., fine. After we've relaxed that group of muscles we will then move to the muscles of the right biceps, and I'll ask you to tense these muscles by pushing your elbow down against the arm of the chair. You should be able to get a feeling of tension in the biceps without involving the muscles in the lower arm and hand. O.K., can you feel tension there now? . . . All right, now after we've completed the relaxation of the right hand and lower arm and the right biceps we'll move over to the muscles of the left hand and left lower arm and tense and relax them in the same way as we did on the right side. We'll also tense and relax the muscles of the left biceps just as we did the right biceps.

After we've relaxed the arms and hands, we'll relax the muscles of the face, and . . . we're going to divide the facial muscles into 3 groups: first the muscles in the forehead area (the upper part of the face), then the muscles in the central part of the face (the upper part of the cheeks and the nose), and finally the lower part of the face (the jaws and the lower part of the cheeks). We'll begin with the muscles in the upper part of the face, and I'll ask you to tense these muscles by lifting the eyebrows just as high as you can and getting tension in the forehead and up into the scalp region. Can you feel that tension now?

O.K., fine. Now we'll move down to the muscles in the central part of the face and in order to tense these muscles I'll ask you to squint your eyes very tightly and at the same time wrinkle up your nose and get tension through the central part of the face. Can you feel the tension there in the upper part of the cheeks and through the eyes now? O.K., good. Next we'll tense the muscles in the lower part of the face and to do this I'll ask you to bite your teeth together and pull the corners of your mouth back. You should feel tension all through the lower part of the face and the jaw. Can you feel the tension in this area now?

Fine. After we've completed the facial muscles we'll move on to relax the muscles of the neck and in order to do this I'm going to ask you to pull your chin downward toward your chest and at the same time try to prevent it from actually touching the chest . . . That is, I want you to *counterpose* the muscles in the front part of the neck against those of the back part of the neck. You should feel just a little bit of shaking or trembling in these muscles as you tense them. Can you feel that now?

O.K., fine. We'll then move to the muscles of the chest, the shoulder and the upper back. We're going to combine quite a few muscles here and I'll ask you to tense these muscles by taking a deep breath, holding it, and at the same time pulling the shoulder blades together; that is, pull the shoulders back and try to make the shoulder blades touch. You should feel significant tension in the chest, the shoulders and the upper back. Can you feel this tension now? O.K., fine.

Now we'll move on to the muscles of the abdomen and in order to tense the muscles in this region, I'm going to ask you to make your stomach hard; just tense it up as though you were going to hit yourself in the stomach. You should feel a good deal of tension and tightness in the stomach area now. Can you feel that tension? O.K., fine.

After relaxing the muscles in the stomach area, we'll then move on to the muscles of the legs and feet, and we'll begin with the right upper leg, the right thigh, and I'll ask you to tense the muscles of the right upper leg by counterposing the one large muscle on top of the leg with the two smaller ones underneath; you should be able to feel that large muscle on top get quite hard. Can you feel that now? O.K., good . . .

We'll then move to the muscles of the left upper leg and tense and relax those muscles just as we did on the right side, then the muscles of the left lower leg, again using the same procedure as we used on the right side, and finally the left foot, tensing it and relaxing it just as we did on the other side.

O.K., fine. Now there are some points I would like to make about this procedure before we begin. I'm going to be asking you to pay very careful attention to the feelings of relaxation that appear in the various muscle groups and since we'll be starting with the right hand and the right lower arm, I'm going to be using that as a reference point against which to compare the next muscle group. So, for example, when we're working on the right biceps I'll ask you a question like 'Does the right biceps feel as relaxed as the right hand and right lower arm?' Thus as we go through this procedure I will be asking for comparative judgements on your part so that we can be assured that each muscle group gets as deeply relaxed as the one prior to it.

Another very important point to remember is that I will expect you to release the tension that you build up in these muscle groups immediately upon my cue. Please don't let the tension dissipate gradually. For example, when you have been tensing the muscles in the right hand and right lower arm, I'll ask you to relax, and when I do, I'd like you to completely and immediately release all the tension that's present in the right hand and lower arm. Do not gradually open the hand; let all the tension go at the same time.

You can see that the first session is quite lengthy. It takes perhaps forty-five minutes to go through all of this, though sessions get shorter as you get used to the exercises. Once completely relaxed you can spend ten minutes or so just basking in the feeling of relaxation before the therapist starts counting backwards from four to one. On the count of four, you start to move your legs and feet. On three, it's the arms and hands; on two the head and neck, and finally on the count of one, you slowly open your eyes, as the therapist says, 'feeling quite calm and relaxed, very pleasantly relaxed, just as if you'd had a brief nap'.

Between sessions at the therapist's office, clients are encouraged to practise at home twice a day for fifteen to twenty minutes. They do so lying on a reclining chair or on the bed, at least an hour after eating a meal, at a time when they are not likely to be interrupted and when they don't feel any time pressure. Early mornings, after work or just before going to bed are all suggested.

Even Type B clients might find this whole process with its sixteen separate muscle groups a bit elaborate. But fortunately, once the individual exercises have been mastered, the process can be telescoped. At first, telescoping is from sixteen groups down to seven. To quote Bernstein and Borkovec again:

... The original sixteen groups are combined as follows:

The muscles of the dominant arm are tensed and relaxed as a single group; thus the hand, lower arm and biceps muscles are combined ... perhaps the easiest procedure is to ask the client to hold the arm out in front of him/her with the elbow bent at about 45 degrees and make a fist, thus tensing not only the muscles of the hand and lower arm, but also the biceps at the same time ...

The muscles of the nondominant arm constitute the second group and are tensed and relaxed in the same way as was group 1.

The next group in the sequence combines the three ... facial muscle groups ... Thus the client should be asked to raise the eyebrows (or frown), squint the eyes, wrinkle up the nose, bite down, and pull the corners of the mouth back. This should produce tension all through the facial area ...

The fourth muscle group is identical to the group employed in the sixteen-group procedure: the neck and throat. This group is tensed just as before.

The fifth muscle group involves combination of the

chest, shoulders, upper back, and abdomen . . . the client should be asked to take a deep breath, hold it, and pull the shoulder blades back and together, while at the same time making the stomach hard (. . . pulling it in or pushing it out).

The muscles of the dominant thigh, calf, and foot constitute the sixth group of muscles . . . the client should be asked to lift the leg off the chair very slightly while pointing the toes and turning the foot inward . . .

The procedure employed for the seventh group (the nondominant thigh, calf, and foot) is identical to that used for group 6.

Finally, the seven muscle groups are combined into just four.

The first of the four groups consists of the muscles of the left and right arms, hands, and biceps. They are combined into one group and are tensed at the same time . . . This may mean that the client is either lifting both arms off the chair and bending them at the elbows or resting them on the chair and making a fist in both hands.

The second group is made up of the muscles of the face and neck. In order to get tension throughout this area, the client should be asked to tense all of the facial muscles while at the same time employing the tension procedure for the neck.

The third muscle group in this procedure includes the muscles of the chest, shoulders, back, and abdomen. There is no change from the seven-group stage.

The final group . . . consists of the muscles of both the left and right upper leg, calf, and foot, and again requires that the client simply combine the tension procedures he had been using in tensing each leg separately . . . If there is any danger that tensing both legs at the same time will cause the client to lose balance and slip out of the chair, the therapist should allow the client to continue tensing one leg at a time, thus creating a five-group technique.

Once the client has learned to achieve deep relaxation using four muscle groups, the relaxation procedure should last less than ten minutes.

The learning sequence for the different patterns involves the sixteen muscle groups for the first three sessions (including the homework in between); the seven muscle groups for the next two, then the four muscle groups for sessions six and seven.

Still lengthy? Perhaps. But this learning of the 'standard' exercises is really only the beginning and life gets simpler once you've mastered the basic skill. The trick is to make it portable and the most important lesson that the therapist can teach his client is how he can relax on exactly those occasions when his tension is about to suddenly increase. For the middle manager, for example, life is full of such moments – unlocking his car to face the drive to work; walking into the office to be told that the managing director wants to see him; scanning the post for problem mail; sitting down to a meeting with his less-than-perfect staff. And of course it happens every time the phone rings. So often has the bad news coming down the phone knotted his stomach that now, like one of Pavlov's dogs, he starts to react as soon as he hears the bell.

One way of dealing with these hassling moments is with *cue-controlled* relaxation. Once you are completely relaxed in his office, the therapist asks you to concentrate on your breathing, to feel and listen to your breaths. Then, each time you breathe out, you say some short calming word to yourself like 'relax', or 'control' or even 'calm' itself. You do this twenty or more times during the session and then repeatedly as part of your home practice. When a client feels that the cue-word has become firmly linked to the feeling of deep relaxation, he goes back mentally to the office and the therapist has him imagine some situation that usually arouses his anxiety – perhaps the thought of something he forgot to do. But instead of leaping up to do it, he uses his cue-word to produce the feeling of relaxation that lessens his anxiety. Another imaginary problem is confronted, then another, each more disturbing than the one before, and on each occasion instead of a pounding heart, a sudden dryness in the mouth and a tightness in the stomach, the cue-word is used to make him relax. Some therapists don't use a word at all. They simply have the client breathe in deeply and slowly when he is completely relaxed and so teach him to link his breathing with the feeling of deep relaxation. He then confronts a series of increasingly difficult, imaginary problems, and uses his breathing to cue his relaxation each time.

Once you've dealt with these situations in your head, you are ready for the problems of real life. As soon as you feel the tell-tale signs that mean you are likely to start reacting (and remember, the fight-or-flight response gets us to anticipate the problem, often before it appears) then you use your word or your breathing to stop yourself from taking off. After a while, you become able to *predict* situations that are likely to make your heart rate and blood pressure shoot up before they ever occur – perhaps walking from your desk to the meeting room, or looking up the phone number of someone you have to confront. These are exactly the times to recall that feeling of deep relaxation and to recreate the feeling by using the cue that you may originally have been shown, but then largely taught yourself.

One thing is certain, you have to start relaxing the very moment you feel the unease. If you delay even for a few seconds your sympathetic system releases enough noradrenaline to keep your heart racing for perhaps half an hour. That doesn't mean hitting the panic button, thinking, 'Oh God, I'm tensing again.' Nothing could get you tense quicker. It does mean listening to your body and learning to recognize its very early feelings of distress and the situations that can turn them on. There may be many of them. A day at work, for example, may be one long series of hassles.

Just how well does all this relaxation actually work? Is it really worth the trouble of learning, either with a teacher or on your own? It works well for anxiety but that's not the overdriver's problem. What we want to know is whether it really does stop sudden surges in blood pressure. Unfortunately, being able to follow your blood pressure during the course of the working day at the office or the factory is still a major project, whether you use an arm cuff or a line inserted directly into an artery. So not many studies of arousal in the workplace, using relaxation as well, seem to have been done so far.

What we do have are encouraging reports about the way that regular relaxation reduces blood pressure over a period of time. Obviously, the greatest interest is in mild hypertensives. To bring their pressures down without drugs would be of enormous value for the twenty-five million or so living in the United States alone. So that's where most of the research effort has been put so far. It doesn't answer the question of controlling the hot responder whose casual pressure may not be raised. But it points in that direction.

For example, Stuart Agras and the Stanford Group wondered whether the pressures of essential hypertensives who were already receiving drugs could be brought down further by teaching them to relax. Ten such patients were taught progressive relaxation, including taking a deep breath and thinking the word 'relax' as they let it out. They did their homework between classes as well, using a set of tape-recorded instructions. They learned the technique over five half-hourly sessions. At the end of the last one they showed an average systolic fall of 14 mm Hg – a very respectable reduction, which was still maintained six months later.

Eleven other patients who also continued on their drugs received warm, enthusiastic and supportive advice from a therapist about how to deal with tense situations, though he didn't give them any instructions in relaxation. At the end of their five sessions, half the group said they *knew* that their pressures had come down, and thanked him warmly. But they were wrong. They had hardly shifted, although they did show some fall during the following five months, presumably as the counsellor's advice started to get through. You need to believe, but belief on its own isn't enough. There's more to relaxation than an act of faith.

But perhaps all the training simply teaches patients to bring their pressures down while it's actually being measured. What happens the rest of the time? To answer that, the Stanford researchers brought five hypertensives into the hospital, and measured their blood pressures frequently over the course of a 'run-in' day, during three days of relaxation training and on the day after. Pressures fell as a result of training, particularly at night. And they were lower on the nights after relaxation than on the other nights, even when the patients were asleep. So the relaxation effect was working even when they didn't know that they were being examined.

To look at the effect that relaxation has on hypertensives during their working day, they had forty-two of them (mostly on medication) wear a blood pressure monitor from eight in the morning until five at night. They had to blow up the cuff every twenty minutes and pressures were recorded automatically. After the first recording day at work, nineteen of them were given eight half-hourly sessions of relaxation training, including instruction on how to relax by scanning their muscles and letting any tension go. They also had regular home practice in which they relaxed while listening to specially produced cassettes.

Nine weeks later they went through the same work-day

measurements. Their average blood pressures at the end of training were 8 mm systolic and 5 mm diastolic lower than they had been at the start. A similar group of hypertensives (also mostly on drugs) who had received no training in how to relax also went through the same measurements on two days, nine weeks apart. But their on-the-job pressures showed no change at all. Regular relaxation seemed to be the key to bringing it down. The Stanford Group concluded that while it may not be a substitute for drugs, it might certainly help to reduce the amount of medication needed by treated hypertensives every day.

An even more detailed look at the value of relaxation for hypertensives was recently conducted in Heidelberg, West Germany. It comes closer than most to treating the overdriver's particular problem. Dr D. Kallinke and his colleagues realized, more than many other physicians have, that relaxation should be taught as a basic coping skill, a technique that can be used in a wide variety of life situations. To introduce their group of over a hundred male hypertensives to this idea, they had them record their blood pressures in many different circumstances. After a dozen casual measurements taken in the clinic, they went out with their blood pressure machines and recorded their own levels three times a day for a week. They kept diaries too, to see what they were doing at the time.

When they came back to the clinic the doctor went through the records with them. He pointed out how some of their biggest rises occurred during disputes with colleagues, while some of their lowest levels were recorded during quiet weekends with the family. They had laboratory tests as well, doing mental arithmetic under time pressure and being subjected to an hour-long interview about life and its problems. Blood pressures were measured during these sessions and each man's pattern of reactions was played back to him.

Once he had come to realize how his pressure responded to outside demands, and to the way that he tried to cope with them, each patient was given twelve sessions of relaxation training. He was also taught ways of coping with situations that were likely to put his pressure up. He was encouraged to use relaxation and calm reflection to deal with them, rather than his usual pattern which only made things worse.

Many of these hypertensives showed great differences between casual pressures measured in the clinic and pressures measured at home. Self measurements were on average 13/8 mm Hg lower than clinic pressures, but both showed an enormous range. In extreme cases, self-measured systolics varied during the day by more than 70 mm and diastolics by more than 50. During the interview about their life and work problems, more than half the patients had rises of 20/10 or more. Most of the increases occurred when they talked about the competition they felt at work and about their reactions to their subordinates and superiors. Discussions about deadlines and job responsibility sent their levels up too.

The effects of the relaxation training were encouraging. Casual pressures taken after they had learned to relax were about 20/10 mm Hg lower than before, and some of this improvement was still found twelve months later. Nor did it seem to matter whether the training had been given individually or in groups. Both seemed equally good.

Unfortunately, the effects on blood pressure measured while the patient was being provoked were 'much less impressive'. When the laboratory tests were run after they had been through the training, the responses were certainly reduced. But the fall was only 8/5 mm Hg, and the self-measured pressures taken during the normal day were down by only 5/2. The research group don't say so, but I suspect that's at least partly because the feeling of relaxation wasn't being switched on either fast or often enough. When you're suddenly taken off guard, it is all too easy to react the way that you've always done.

Although some of these German hypertensives didn't show much variation in their blood pressure, those who did so belonged to two different groups. The first were suffering from obvious life events like marital crises, bereavement or unemployment. Some of them were permanently overworked or extremely competitive. What they needed was specific counselling about how to handle their specific problems. But for the others (the majority) blood pressure rose in response to a whole range of situations in both their private and their professional lives. What they needed was to learn more general methods of problem-solving that could be applied to many different events, as and when they came along.

We shall see how this type of problem-solving can be taught, just as relaxation can. But because of his chronic time-urgency you might think that progressive relaxation, with cues or without, and problem-solving as well would be too time-consuming for the Type A to even consider. At first glance, he might be more tempted by biofeedback.

There was tremendous excitement among psychologists in the 1960s when it was realized that some of the body's so-called 'involuntary' functions, like heart rate and blood pressure, weren't involuntary at all. Previously they had believed that activities driven by the sympathetic or parasympathetic systems couldn't be brought under conscious control. Your heart beat fast or slow whatever you might want it to do.

But experiments first with animals then with human volunteers showed that this wasn't so. You could control your pulse rate or your systolic pressure if you were given information about what was happening. So, for example, an electronic device measuring your heart rate turned it into a sound played over a loudspeaker, or your blood pressure was measured and the level was displayed as a line on a TV screen. In other words, information about your body's functions that you couldn't assess easily (or at all) for yourself, was fed back to you in a form that you could easily see or hear. To change your own internal state, you had to concentrate on making the pitch of the feedback sound higher or lower, or making the line on the video display rise or fall.

Many people found that they could. With training, their pulses or pressures could be shifted up or down, their levels of muscle tension could be reduced or their brain waves changed, all in response to the biofeedback display. It seemed that the new dawn of self-control had finally arrived. Few of the subjects could say how they actually did it. They stumbled by trial and error on whatever sense or feeling it was that shifted the display. But having found it they learned to switch it on at will. To encourage them in the laboratory sessions they were often rewarded, either with praise or money (or slides of *Playboy* centrefolds in one case). But generally the satisfaction of just being able to exert such control was enough of an incentive.

Recent research has shown biofeedback to have an advantage over relaxation as a way of keeping blood pressure down, at least in the laboratory. It works well in situations where you are being hassled, a problem that cue-induced relaxation hasn't reliably solved as yet. For example, Dr Andrew Steptoe of St George's Hospital in London asked two groups of volunteers to try lowering their blood pressure either by feedback or relaxation. First they did so in a quiet restful environment, and both methods worked. Then they were asked to keep it low while being forced to perform a task that demanded their attention. They heard a number of sounds, and as each was played they had to respond by pressing one of four buttons to indicate which sound it was.

Faced with this extra involvement, the relaxation group weren't able to stop their blood pressures from rising, but the feedback group carried on as though nothing had happened. A similar thing happened when both had to solve mental arithmetic problems while controlling their pressures at the same time. All the volunteers showed a rise in blood pressure when they first heard the questions, but it fell back to normal much more quickly for those practising feedback rather than relaxation.

So why hasn't biofeedback brought the new dawn, and why do many of those who have spent years working on it now feel some sense of disappointment about its potential for getting blood pressures down? The main reason is that although many people can produce quite large falls while they are hooked up to some complex feedback machine, the learning pattern doesn't easily carry over into the world outside. Out in the street or in the office, without the feedback display in front of us, we seem much less able to produce the same results. But the overdriver, like the hypertensive, needs something he can carry around, preferably inside him, to use whenever he feels the need. Biofeedback, it seems, isn't it.

But since both can lower blood pressure separately, is there any prospect of using biofeedback and relaxation together? And if the feedback were made as simple as possible, would that help? According to Dr Michael S. Glasgow at the Baltimore City Hospital and his colleagues, Drs Bernard T. Engel and Kenneth R. Gaarder, it might. To compare feedback and relaxation, they recruited ninety hypertensive volunteers. Since they knew only too well how blood pressures can vary during the day, they gave each one a pressure machine with a large easy-to-read dial. After teaching them how to take their own pressures they sent them off for a month to record their levels three times a day – in the morning, during the afternoon and at night. At the end of that time, patient and doctor went through the month of records to see how the pressures varied and when they were highest. Greatest pressures were usually recorded between about noon and 4.00 p.m.

With this 'baseline' pattern established, the volunteers were taught either relaxation or biofeedback. Those in the progressive relaxation group had only a single lesson on how to do it – far less than most psychologists would recommend. They were then asked to practise ten-minute relaxation sessions as often in the day as possible, particularly when they thought their pressures were likely to be raised. During the first month they were to use the method as they'd learned it. But later they were also told to try to 'develop a sense of the feeling of relaxation', and to try relaxing in response to cues from outside. For example, they were to switch on the relaxation at traffic signals or during breaks at work.

The feedback procedure was especially clever. Instead of a large electronic device, the patient used the pressure machine itself to give them their signals. They blew up the cuff and as it deflated they listened through the stethoscope for the first gurgling sounds that represent the systolic pressure level. As the cuff deflated further they listened for the point at which the sounds disappeared – the diastolic level. They recorded them both. The feedback training was to let the cuff pressure fall to where the systolic sounds were heard last time, and to try to prevent them this time round. If patients were successful they would drop the cuff pressure by another 2 mm then try again, until they reached the point where the systolic sounds couldn't be held back any longer.

They did this for a month, several times a day. The following month they were encouraged to 'develop a sense of the feedback response' to try to identify the internal feelings that went with a reducing systolic pressure. In the third month they were to practise with and without the machine and to try to lower their pressures on cue. Some patients then spent another three months (six months in all) doing the same thing again. But others were switched over, from relaxation to feedback or vice versa, for the second half of the trial.

A long study like this generated a lot of results. The most obvious and encouraging was the way that pressures measured by the patients themselves in the afternoons came down by some 5–10 mm Hg during the treatment. The biggest falls were in those who practised feedback for the first three months, then relaxation for the second. The Baltimore group suggest that feedback may be helping to relax those arteries in the body that have become constricted, with a resulting rise in blood pressure. The relaxation on the other hand, was thought to reduce the output of blood from the heart, which also raises the pressure, especially when it is being forced down narrowed arteries.

Whether the two approaches work this way or not, the results do show the value of a home blood pressure machine, both as a monitor and as a source of feedback. Indeed, Engel and his colleagues even suggest a 'stepped care program' for mild hypertensives, like that used by the HDFP, but this one using a behavioural approach instead of the increasing use of drugs.

Borderline cases (those with diastolics less than 105 mm Hg or those receiving diuretics alone) should monitor their own pressures three times daily for a month. If they stay in the range that their physicians consider acceptable, they should go on doing so and he should check them only at six-monthly intervals. If not, they should try feedback for three months, and if that doesn't bring them into the acceptable range they should practise relaxation for a further three months before patient and doctor finally agree that drugs (or more drugs) are required.

So feedback has its uses, as long as the gadgetry is kept simple. It may bring pressures down and if you really can learn to develop a 'sense of the feedback response' to switch on when required, it may help those of you who are hot responders to learn how to cool your outbursts. At the very least, it can help you to monitor the success you may be having with other approaches, which is exactly how it has been used in the most successful treatment yet devised for reducing blood pressure without drugs.

10. From Relaxation to Meditation

It is little more than ten years since Dr Chandra Patel, a general practitioner in Croydon, first surprised many physicians with the success that she could achieve in lowering blood pressures using a combination of biofeedback and what she called 'yoga relaxation'. Since that time many other research groups have tried to do the same, and indeed, the interest developed by Stuart Agras and his colleagues at Stanford was largely the result of having read Chandra Patel's work.

Her best-known early study involved a group of thirty-four 'moderate' hypertensive patients in a general practice. Nearly all of them were taking drugs, but even so their average pressures were about 170/100. They were divided into two groups – one to be treated now, one later. After attending her surgery on three separate days to measure their 'baseline' blood pressures as accurately as possible, the group who were to be treated straight away were shown films and slides explaining what high blood pressure is and why it is dangerous. They were then introduced to the idea of bodily relaxation and self-control and they were also told about biofeedback. Then they were encouraged to ask any questions about their own particular situations, and how all this might apply to them.

Having been fully prepared in this way, patients reclined on a chair or a couch and were taught a way of relaxing completely. Then having relaxed, they learned a form of meditation. At the same time, they were connected to a biofeedback machine which either measured how moist their hands were or whether their muscles were still tense. Sympathetic arousal makes your palms sweat – often not much, not even enough for you to notice – but quite enough to be detected electrically. The biofeedback information was converted into a sound, and as the hypertensives became more relaxed, so the sound fell in pitch. The feedback let them know how well they were doing.

Patients came to these thirty-minute relaxation sessions twice a week for six weeks. For the first fifteen minutes they went through the relaxation routine. In the second half of each session they practised their meditation. They were also encouraged to do the same at home twice a day and to try to incorporate the relaxation procedure into their daily lives.

Blood pressures were measured before and after every session during the six-week period that they regularly saw the doctor. They were then followed for another three months to see how their pressures might change when they were simply practising by themselves. The changes were striking. Between the first session and the last they showed an average fall of 26 mm Hg systolic and 15 mm diastolic. So the treatment looked very promising, but what was it due to? Was it simply the result of intensive interest and attention on the doctor's part?

I said that Dr Patel's patients were divided at the start into two groups. Only one group was taught relaxation to begin with. The others, who attended the same number of sessions, were asked to relax for themselves as best they could, but they weren't told how, nor did they receive any feedback, and their own relaxation wasn't nearly as good. At the end of the twelve sessions their pressures were down, but only by an average of 9/4 mm Hg (I say 'only' though many physicians would be delighted to do as well). So being in a trial at all was having some effect. It always does. But the relaxation was producing benefits of its own and to prove that this was true, Chandra Patel took the seventeen hypertensives who had so far received no active treatment and put them through exactly the same twelve-week programme. By the end, their pressures had dropped by an average of 28/15, just like the first group. The treatment was having a real effect.

So what are these relaxation exercises that can produce such striking falls in blood pressure? They are based on yoga, a Hindu religious tradition that has been practised in India for many centuries. But to learn this type of relaxation you don't have to believe in any religious or spiritual system. You can think of it purely as a technique.

Once the patient is reclining on the chair or the couch (at home often on the bed), Dr Patel instructs him (or her) to make contact with every part of the body. Her method is similar in some ways to progressive muscle relaxation, but rather than tensing followed by release, it simply concentrates on scanning your muscles and relaxing whatever tension you find there already – something progressive relaxers are taught to do at a later stage. But it is a concentration on breathing that makes her approach so obviously a part of yoga. In the yogic system (as Patel explains) there is believed to be an energy or force (Prana) in the air, and breathing exercises are designed to pass the force into and through your body. But she also explains that you don't have to believe in anything except oxygen for the benefits to work.

Having achieved this quite deep level of relaxation, you can either simply enjoy it for its own sake or, as her patients did, go on to the next stage which is one of meditation. Your senses are withdrawn from outside distractions. Your mind passively concentrates on some special focus of attention (in this case a word) and it may even start to approach a different level of consciousness. However, it isn't necessary to know much about the long history of these exercises or the philosophy behind them for the blood pressure effects to work. Indeed, Dr Patel herself says that 'whether any of the patients reaches anywhere near a meditative state is highly questionable. But whatever mental calm he can get is useful.'

The question, of course, is whether the mental calm that you learn in the doctor's surgery and practise in the quiet of your bedroom can be useful to you in your car, in the street or at work, where problems are coming at you from all sides. Far from reserving it for the quiet moments, she suggests that you practise many times a day, in just those situations that get you aroused. Obviously that doesn't mean the whole relaxation procedure, much less the meditation. Instead, patients are taught how to recall that inner feeling of what it is like to be relaxed – a feeling learned at a quieter time – and to switch the feeling on when it is needed. Like many other therapists, Chandra Patel also advises her patients to stick a small paper disc (usually red) on their watch and on the telephone. Others suggest sticking one on your steering wheel, and on the lift button – all of them objects that normally increase your arousal. But when you catch sight of the disc, the opposite happens. The red dot is your cue to relax, if only for a moment.

And does it work in real life? Is it possible to keep your blood pressure down when you're being hassled? Patel's experiments suggest that it is. She measured the blood pressures of a group of middle-aged hypertensives who were asked to perform two arousing tasks in the laboratory. First they climbed twenty-five times on and off a box. Later they stuck their hand into a bucket of ice-cold water. Their blood pressure responses were measured on both occasions.

They were then given the six-week training programme of relaxation, meditation and biofeedback, and the tests were repeated. Their responses were compared with their own reactions before the training and with a second group of hypertensives who had attended the clinic just as often but who had tried to relax on their own. And by comparing the size of the blood pressure rises and the time it took for pressures to fall back to normal, it was clear that the trained patients nearly always did better. So as well as reducing pressure over a period of weeks or months, the relaxation training also seemed to bring their short-term reactions more under control, in these situations at least.

Relaxation has other benefits too, that weren't expected when Chandra Patel began. It can be used on a large scale, and it can work on more than blood pressure. In the late 1970s, she and her co-workers decided to take their relaxation training into industry. Over one thousand, two hundred employees in a British manufacturing firm were invited to have their risk factors screened and 20 per cent were found to have two or more of their risks increased. That is to say, they had blood pressures of 140/90 or more, or cholesterols of at least 240 mg/100 ml, or else they smoked ten or more cigarettes a day. They were eligible for a treatment trial if they had two risk factors raised out of three.

About two hundred of them agreed to take part in an eight-week programme to see whether their risks could be reduced. They all of them received an individual explanation about the purpose of the study, and they all got literature on how to change their dietary fats and their smoking habits. In addition, about half of them attended a series of weekly, hour-long group sessions where six or eight at a time were taught breathing, relaxation and meditation. This time the instructions were on a pre-recorded cassette. All the volunteers were hooked up to a machine that measured hand sweating, and the information was fed back to each one of them individually, so that they could see (or rather hear) how they were doing. Each one was encouraged to practise what he had learned in his everyday life, and each was lent an instruction cassette with which to practise at home.

Risk factors were measured at the end of the eight weeks and again at eight months to look for long-term changes. Those who had been taught to relax were compared with a similar group who had the initial briefing and the educational literature but who hadn't had the relaxation training. Both at eight weeks and eight months the average fall in blood pressure was about 14/7 mm Hg for all the subjects in the relaxation group, and for those who had raised pressures at the start the fall was even greater – about 20/10. As you'd expect, blood pressures fell in the untreated group as well, but not by nearly so much.

There were other changes too. In those volunteers whose cholesterols had been raised, the relaxation training produced an average drop of 35 mg/100 ml after eight weeks. At least, there seemed no other explanation for the fall. Changes in weight and in diet were both measured and neither could account for it. Presumably it resulted from a general lowering of arousal, as we saw with Friedman's accountants. At the same time, about 10 per cent of the treated group stopped smoking over the eight weeks, and had still stopped at eight months, while only half as many as the untreated group did so.

If these risk factor reductions could be applied to British men as a whole (and if reducing risk factors also means reducing the death rate) then they might produce a fall in CHD mortality of about 20 per cent. They measure up well to the intervention results obtained in places like North Karelia, even though Patel's emphasis was on relaxation, with dietary and smoking advice coming further down the list.

So it seems that a relaxation programme linked with biofeedback and meditation can produce some striking falls in blood pressure and in cholesterol too. The instructions can be taught off a tape and the whole package can be used by large groups of people. But will meditation on its own without the feedback have any effect? Some people have certainly claimed so. Indeed, transcendental meditation (TM) has been marketed on a huge scale as a treatment for many different physical and psychological problems. It has not lived up to its promise, and many of those who originally took it up dropped it again just as quickly. And that's a pity. Because despite the exaggerations and the inflated optimism, despite the fact that scientific investigations have stripped it of many of its claims, TM and its more 'secular' variations still have a lot to offer.

Transcendental meditation was brought from India to the West by Maharishi Mahesh Yogi in the late 1950s. By the late 1970s over half a million people in the United States had been taught the technique and even in Britain initiates numbered a hundred thousand. The practice of TM involves sitting quietly and allowing your mind to contemplate a particular word or 'mantra'. By so doing, your attention, which is normally engaged in many different activities at the same time, becomes focused in one direction. Other thoughts and feelings become secondary and you enter a state of 'passive awareness'. You know what is going on, both inside and outside your body, but your mind becomes detached, observing it all, but separated from it. Rather than concentrating on individual thoughts, TM students are encouraged to make mental contact with the source from which all their thoughts originate. It's not unlike Chandra Patel's approach, and indeed, she originally described her own procedure as 'a type of transcendental meditation'. Where she parts company with the TM movement is in the ballyhoo that goes with it.

The mantra is given by the teacher to each student during his initiation and he promises never to reveal it. Patel lets you choose your own. The initiation ceremony in TM also has a quasi-religious flavour that reflects its origins in the Hindu scriptures and has attracted criticism from two sides. On the one hand are those who have spent many years studying Hinduism. They suggest that what the Maharishi brought to the West is only a small part of a rich and complex system, and even that has been distorted and packaged for Western consumption. On the other are those who feel that religious overtones are simply unnecessary for the practice of what is, after all, a simple routine procedure, a method that can be followed by anyone and that doesn't require any belief system at all – except perhaps the belief that it will work. This natural suspicion combined with the claims of the TM movement to be able to bring harmony to the world, means that for many people the whole organization has simply discredited itself.

For example, in 1979 I was invited to the inaugural session of my local 'City Parliament of the Age of Enlightenment'. The invitation explained how His Holiness Maharishi Mahesh Yogi had founded the World Government of the Age of Enlightenment to 'raise the level of world consciousness, create an ideal society and bring invincibility and all possibilities to every nation'. Looking out at me were the photographs of eleven well-groomed young men, the Ministers of the World Government for Great Britain. They included a Minister for the Development of Consciousness, for Prosperity and Progress, for Health and Immortality, and there was even a Ministry of All Possibilities. The invitation further explained how, during 1978, the Governors of the Age of Enlightenment successfully 'calmed down violence and restored peace in the five most troubled areas of the world' by their daily practice of the TM programme – an event which I must have missed.

It would be too easy to ridicule the stunning naivety on which the whole movement seems to be based, let alone the much-publicized claim that those who follow (and pay for) the advanced TM programme can learn to levitate. And it would take me too far from the question of what meditation can do for the overdriver. The reason why TM attracted attention in medical circles wasn't because of the Age of Enlightenment. It was because of the publication in the early 1970s of a series of results describing the bodily changes that apparently occurred as the result of practising it regularly. They were written by Mr Robert Keith Wallace of the University of California at Irvine (now Dr Wallace of the Maharishi University at Fairfield, Iowa), and Dr Herbert Benson of the Boston City Hospital and Harvard Medical School.

The two researchers carried out a whole series of measurements on thirty-six volunteers who had been practising TM on average for a couple of years. The tests were performed when they were sitting quietly with their eyes open, and then when they were meditating with their eyes closed. During meditation the amount of oxygen that the subjects consumed was reported to fall by nearly 20 per cent – twice the fall that happens during sleep. Their rate of breathing out carbon dioxide also fell as indeed did their breathing rate itself, suggesting that the whole of their body's metabolism was slowing down. Pulse rates were reduced and skin resistance rose, both measures of decreased sympathetic arousal. Even more striking was the change reported in their brain wave patterns – an increase of 'slow alpha' waves – thought to be associated with a state of passive mental alertness. So dramatic were these changes when taken together that Wallace and Benson described TM as a 'wakeful hypometabolic state', and Wallace in his later writings went so far as to describe transcendental meditation as a 'fourth state of consciousness', distinct from waking, sleeping and dreaming.

Such hefty claims naturally produced a critical response from other research teams. A group led by Dr P. B. C. Fenwick of St Thomas's Hospital in London examined meditators, from novices to experienced teachers, and found that during meditation their oxygen intake did indeed go down, but not by nearly as much as the American studies had found. Nor was there any evidence that meditation reduced the body's metabolic rate below that resulting from simple muscle relaxation. As to the brain wave changes, they were like those seen during the early stages of falling asleep. In short, 'No support was found for the idea that transcendental meditation is a fourth state of consciousness.'

Other researchers went further. One group actually suggested that meditators spend part of their meditation asleep – and quite deeply asleep at that. They questioned whether the benefits of TM were simply the result of getting extra sleep during the daytime. And Dr Jonathan C. Smith, then at the University of Michigan, suggested that it might not be sleeping, but simply sitting quietly twice a day, confident that TM would work, that caused its beneficial effects.

During his week of training, attempts are made to build up the aspiring meditator's confidence in the method by a number of introductory lectures, in which the rationale of meditation is explained, scientific results relating to TM (like those of Wallace and Benson) are reviewed, and any questions or doubts are answered. Smith decided to recreate this air of confidence to boost a treatment method of his own called, imposingly enough, 'periodic somatic inactivity' or PSI. It consisted of sitting absolutely still with your eyes closed twice a day – just that, nothing else. Would-be initiates received two introductory lectures in which the technique was introduced to them as 'an immensely credible cure for most forms of psychopathology'. It had its own initiation ceremony, and its own set of scientific results that students had described to them. PSI was taught by an enthusiastic undergraduate teacher who had been supplied with a 71-page book containing answers to 'frequently asked questions' about the method. His own belief and dedication to PSI were complete.

But it was all quite bogus – a totally made-up system designed to create the same expectations as TM, something that even the teacher didn't know until much later. The important feature was that it worked. The anxiety that it was used to treat improved with either TM or PSI. Both methods were better than giving no treatment at all, but they were no different from each other. With that, Smith reached the inevitable conclusion. Whatever else it may be 'the critical therapeutic component of TM is not the TM exercise . . .'

So why, with all these failures in the past, do I still consider transcendental meditation as a useful way of de-activating the overdriver's arousal? Two reasons. First, despite the claims and counter-claims, TM does have a beneficial effect on blood pressure. And second, it has now been simplified and 'secularized' into a technique that you can learn for yourself in less than an hour.

It was Herbert Benson and his colleagues in Boston who found that TM reduced blood pressure both in borderline hypertensives and in those being treated with drugs. They recruited their volunteers from the Students' International Meditation Society, an organization set up to teach TM at a fee (in the mid-1970s) of $75. Subjects attending the introductory lectures and who knew themselves to be hypertensives, were told the fee would be waived if they would delay learning the technique for six weeks, during which they would have their baseline blood pressures measured. They also agreed that after learning to meditate they would return every few weeks to have their pressures checked again (at times when they weren't actually meditating) to see what effect twenty minutes of meditation twice a day was having on their casual pressures.

In all, twenty-two borderline volunteers were taught to meditate and were followed for about six months. Their average pressure before their initiation was 147/95 mm Hg.

Six months later it had fallen by 7 mm systolic and 4 mm diastolic – falls which the research team admit are small, but still worth having. They also recruited a group of meditating hypertensives whose pressures while on drugs averaged 146/92. As a result of TM they fell by 11/5 mm. Again, the falls were not spectacular, but they raised the possibility of being able to reduce the hypertensive's drug dosage.

Other research groups have done better. Drs Peter Seer and John M. Raeburn of the University of Auckland Medical School in New Zealand, achieved a drop of 20 per cent in systolic pressure and about half as much in diastolic, when unmedicated hypertensives meditated on the mantra 'shyam'. But their meditation was a very practical exercise. The emphasis was put on it being a method of 'self-relaxation', not as anything mystical. Of course, this change in emphasis from the spiritual to the material had already happened before the New Zealand workers began their studies. Indeed, it is probably the biggest contribution that Herbert Benson has made to the whole subject.

In his various research papers, and his most successful book *The Relaxation Response* Benson has traced the similarities that he found in forms of meditation practised in different parts of the world over many centuries. He set out to capture the essence of the process, not, he stresses, as a *substitute* for a spiritual awakening, but rather as a technique that would lend itself to scientific investigation. The result is his own meditation procedure, the so-called *relaxation response*, the instructions for which (as published in the prestigious *New England Journal of Medicine*) go like this:

Sit quietly in a comfortable position. Close your eyes. Deeply relax all your muscles, beginning at your feet and progressing up to your face. Keep them deeply relaxed.

Breathe through your nose. Become aware of your breathing. As you breathe out, say the word 'one' silently to yourself. Continue for 20 minutes. You may open your eyes to check the time, but do not use an alarm. When you have finished, sit quietly for several minutes, at first with closed eyes and later with opened eyes.

Do not worry about whether you are successful in achieving a deep level of relaxation. Maintain a passive attitude and permit relaxation to occur at its own pace. Expect distracting thoughts. When these distracting thoughts occur, ignore them and continue repeating 'one'.

Practice the technic once or twice daily, but not within two hours after a meal, since the digestive processes seem to interfere with elicitation of anticipated changes.

You will be struck by the similarity between Benson's method and that used by Chandra Patel, particularly in putting you into an initial state of relaxation and then developing an awareness of your own breathing. However, Benson's approach is not as detailed. It doesn't require the therapist's voice (either live or on tape) and it is specifically meant for you to learn yourself ('in just five minutes' according to the blurb on the book-jacket).

But can such a simple procedure really have any effect? Yes it can – the same effect as TM apparently. Benson and his colleagues had a group of healthy young volunteers learn the relaxation response simply by reading it off an instruction sheet. After practising for no more than an hour they were asked to produce it in the laboratory while their reactions were being measured. Just as in the TM experiments, their oxygen intake fell by 13 per cent, carbon dioxide output came down by a similar amount and their respiration fell by five breaths a minute while they were practising it, but not when they were just sitting quietly. This time, however, there was no talk of a 'fourth state of consciousness'. This time there was a more solid explanation of the response and how it worked. But before we look at what it is, let's see what evoking the relaxation response can do to normal blood pressures.

Benson's team turned to a large industrial complex in Wilmington, Massachusetts, to discover whether taking regular 'relaxation breaks' during the day would have any effect on the workers' overall performance and sense of well-being. They invited all the employees on a single factory site to volunteer for a study concerned with 'combatting the harmful effects of stress'. More than a hundred did so. They were divided into several groups and after four weeks of 'baseline' measurements, one group of fifty-eight were taught how to produce the relaxation response by attending two or three hour-long training sessions at which they practised relaxation and were encouraged to discuss the experience. A second group were taught to sit quietly with their eyes closed, and the others received no special instructions.

The plan was for the first two groups to spend two fifteen-minute break periods either relaxing or just sitting. One break was to be in the morning, the other in the afternoon. The company set aside a quiet room with comfortable chairs for the purpose, but it was stressed that employees had to take their breaks in their own time, and most of them ended up having at least one of their sessions at home. Those practising the relaxation settled down to an average of about nine sessions a week.

During the eight weeks of the study, the volunteers regularly reported to the company's first-aid room to have their blood pressures taken. They also filled out records that were used to assess their general state of health. For example, one questionnaire measured illness symptoms like headache, nausea or diarrhoea, sleep problems and worry that they might be experiencing, first at the beginning of the study, then again at the end. In the group practising relaxation (but not in any of the others) these symptoms became less common as time went by. Other measures of well-being also tended to be better among the relaxation group, perhaps because 'taking such relaxation breaks may be associated with improvements in one's perception of one's health and performance and in one's self-satisfaction',

But it was the blood pressure results that were of particular interest. Between the first and last readings, pressures in the relaxation group fell by 12/8 mm Hg. That wasn't all due to the response itself. We've seen how blood pressures come down simply by being in a blood pressure study, and volunteers who just sat quietly showed a fall of 7/3. But those employees who didn't do anything, didn't show any fall either. So while just sitting is good, sitting and meditating is better. It's also worth noting that the Wilmington volunteers as a whole weren't hypertensive at all. The average blood pressure in the relaxation group, before they ever learned to relax, was only 120/79 – a pressure that many hypertensives would be very glad to get down to *after* treatment.

Herbert Benson and his colleagues were careful not to go overboard about the results. After all, they were confined to a two-month period. It wasn't possible to say whether they would be maintained with longer practice, let alone whether they would influence the overall rate of sickness or death. All the same, the fact that the response reduced blood pressures even in normotensives meant that 'it might become a most useful component of preventive as well as therapeutic programs'.

And that's where some of us see it in relation to overdrive. As a twice-daily procedure, you practise it first in the morning in preparation for the rest of the day. By having some little time to yourself, by distancing yourself, if only briefly, from the day's forthcoming problems and by giving both your body and your mind a basis of calm from which to operate, you can help yourself to avoid (or at least delay) the first morning blow-up. By practising again later you can reaffirm this sense of calmness and delay the first of the afternoon explosions. In between, you can briefly recapture the 'sense of meditation' as often as you need to. The time investment is minimal, and although a few people who practise meditation for hours experience some emotional disturbance, Benson reports seeing no side-effects at all in people practising the response for ten to twenty minutes twice daily over a five-year period. Indeed, many of his patients have reported it to be a pleasurable experience and meditators in general agree. At least that part of the TM teaching is true.

But I said there was a rationale. So how do all these methods work? What do progressive relaxation or TM or the relaxation response actually do to you? To start with, it's a mistake to lump them all together. Progressive relaxation is a set of purely physical reactions. Your mind is concentrated on your muscle groups, but beyond that it isn't a mental training. By contrast, forms of passive meditation like TM and Benson's method (and there are several others) focus your attention on one specific item – for example your mantra or your feeling of breathing. This eventually brings about a mental change, a change in your awareness, perhaps even a change in the way that you see the world. No such claims can be made for muscle relaxation, and it's unfortunate that Herbert Benson labelled his particular type of *meditation* as the *relaxation* response in the first place. He did so because he believed that deep relaxation and meditation have the same physical effects. He thought they work through the same pathway. In his view they both reverse the fight-or-flight reaction.

Benson has drawn attention several times to the way in which the sympathetic reactions of fight-or-flight can be triggered in experimental animals by stimulating particular areas of the brain. The physical effects of TM or the relaxation response when taken together – reduced oxygen intake and breathing rate, a fall in heart rate and long-term blood pressure – seem to be the very reverse of this aroused sympathetic state. He therefore suggested that these forms of meditation may have an effect on the brain regions which lower the body's level of sympathetic activity.

Drs Bernard C. Glueck and Charles S. Stroebel of the Institute for Living in Hartford, Connecticut, have gone further. They point out that regularly repeating the mantra will set up a repetitive low-frequency input in the brain's speech area. The regular sound vibration becomes translated into electrical activity and so meditators produce a regular firing of nerve cells in this region. But the various parts of the brain are interconnected. The resonant reaction moves 'upwards' to influence the pattern of nerve firing in the higher brain centres – hence the increase in regular alpha rhythm that Wallace and Benson originally reported. But the resonant firing pattern also moves 'downwards' to quieten those brain centres that govern the sympathetic system. So we go from the sound of the mantra to reduced sympathetic arousal in one rather elegant step.

Unfortunately, neither Herbert Benson nor anyone else has so far been able to prove it. As Dr Richard L. Verrier, also of the Harvard Medical School, pointed out at a scientific meeting where I was reporting some data on Benson's behalf, the sympathetic and parasympathetic systems rarely work independently. As the activity of one increases, the effects of the other decline. So it is a mistake to concentrate simply on one – in this case the sympathetic – and the ways in which it might be suppressed.

More recent results from a research group in Cologne, West Germany, led by Dr R. Lang, show how true this is. They put twenty TM teachers through a series of tests that involved either sitting still, exercising or meditating. They found that immediately after meditation the noradrenaline concentrations in their blood plasma, far from being reduced, were actually increased. But at the same time their heart rates had fallen – two effects in opposite directions. What was the explanation? The German team suggest that during meditation, sympathetic activity actually goes up. The fact that meditators are 'sharper' – mentally more vigilant – afterwards also suggests the same thing. However, they believe that the parasympathetic system is activated at the same time to keep the heart rate low – remember what happens in the dentist's chair? So the effects of meditation may be twofold.

Since then, Benson himself has found something similar. Nineteen volunteers at the Beth Israel Hospital in Boston were put through a series of increasingly more strenuous activities, while they had blood samples collected at five-minute intervals. First they simply lay down, while blood was taken for 'baseline' measurements. Then they stood up and gripped a compression spring (like a body-builder's wrist developer) with a third of their maximum grip strength. Finally, they gripped it as hard as they could, and held it there for five minutes – the sort of exercise that makes your arm tremble and your teeth clench tight.

Nine of them were taught the relaxation response and asked to practise it for twenty minutes twice a day for a month. The other ten were simply asked to sit quietly for the same length of time. At the end of the month they came back to the hospital and went through the whole procedure again.

Noradrenaline levels in blood plasma increased dramatically as the tasks got harder. They were four times higher standing up gripping the spring at full pressure than they were lying down. And with those volunteers who had learned the relaxation response and went through the procedure for a second time, their noradrenalines went up even further. On the second occasion there was a sixfold difference between lying down and gripping at full pressure.

Far from a fall in sympathetic activity, Benson's technique had produced an increase. When the 'control' group were taught the relaxation response during the second month and they too came back to be retested, the same thing happened – more noradrenaline than before they had learned it.

Surprising as that was, it was only half the story. Blood pressures and heart rates were measured at the same time. Naturally, both increased as the tasks became more strenuous. But the increase during the second session, after the relaxation practice, was no higher than during the first. If anything, the rise was slightly less, despite the increased noradrenaline which you would expect to increase both.

To the Boston group this implied that more noradrenaline is needed to produce the same rise in heart rate and blood pressure in people who know how to meditate. The reason isn't clear. Perhaps the noradrenaline receptors (remember the beta-receptors that are put out of action by beta-blockers) become less responsive. But so far, that's a long shot. It's difficult to imagine how such a natural beta-blockade could happen. It seems just as likely that the excess noradrenaline hits the receptors but that the parasympathetic system overrides its effects.

What does seem clear is that regular meditation somehow 'disconnects' the sympathetic system from some of its more dangerous consequences. It certainly seems to blunt the blood pressure response, the sort of uncoupling that so far we've only been able to achieve with drugs. It's exactly what the overdriver needs – an easily learned, do-it-yourself exercise, to be practised morning and afternoon, the whole thing taking no more than half an hour a day.

Of course, you may prefer progressive relaxation or a more 'spiritual' form of mantra meditation. You may even prefer biofeedback with a blood pressure machine, if you've got one. For any of these you need a teacher, at least to get you started. But the overdriver I have in mind has no time for tuition. He may have none for the relaxation response either: 'What, half an hour a day, are you kidding? Where am I going to find that sort of time? I'm pushed to the limit as it is.' And it's true. He is. But he doesn't have to be. What he needs to do is to sort out his priorities.

11. Out of Overdrive

'This card might save your life.' So ran an advertisement in the western edition of *Time* magazine one day in 1977. The reply-paid card invited men living around San Francisco who had suffered a coronary to join a research programme. Its object was to stop them from having another, by changing their Type A behaviour.

Meyer Friedman was the driving force behind this project to prevent second heart attacks. Originally planned to involve 1000 men over a period of five years, it is now virtually complete. And it has been a success. Many of the men who were counselled about changing their behaviour managed to do so. As a result, this counselled group showed only half as many reinfarctions as men who received all the latest cardiological advice but were not taught how to modify their Type A behaviour. So striking was the difference between the two groups that the experiment was concluded after not five but only four and a half years. The point had been adequately made.

This Recurrent Coronary Prevention Project (or RCPP, as it came to be known) is the only investigation so far to have successfully modified Type A behaviour and reduced the heart attack rate as a result. Like the WCGS, it is a spectacular achievement, and we will look at it in detail later. Its results will be analysed and argued over for years to come.

But what is there to argue about, if its results are so clear-cut? The controversy will centre around two questions. The first is whether it is possible to change Type A behaviour in men who haven't yet had a coronary. The second is whether the RCPP approach is a feasible way of getting them to do so. The project aimed to produce a fundamental change in many aspects of the sufferer's life. He had to be prepared to revise his whole pattern of behaviour, to re-evaluate what and how he thought, and to examine carefully and *go on* examining how he felt and how his body was reacting in a whole range of situations, both on his own and with other people.

Such a degree of change may be simply too much to hope for in men or women who think of themselves as basically healthy. And Friedman himself doubts whether this degree of commitment to change is likely to be made by anyone who hasn't actually had a heart attack. So the search has been on for the last ten years to find some simpler approach, some acceptable 'treatment package' to save the overdriver from himself before he feels the first pains in his chest.

So far we don't have one. We don't have it because we don't really know how to motivate healthy people to change their behaviour. But worse than that, we're still not sure what particular aspects of overdrive we ought to be aiming at. Is it the Type A's loud, explosive speech, his competitive drive and impatient time-urgency, or his easily aroused anger that we have to try and modify? Probably we have to go for them all. They all seem to carry a risk.

For example, when you start talking, your blood pressure goes up. When you stop it comes down again. For many years, measuring blood pressure in the physician's surgery was a silent ritual. For most of us it still is. The doctor doesn't say anything because he wants you to stay calm, and anyway he's listening to the arterial sounds through the stethoscope. You don't say anything because you're even more anxious to keep calm, and anyway you don't want to distract the doctor's attention. But the arrival of automatic blood pressure recorders that inflate themselves, measure the pressure and give a printed read-out has changed all that. Dr James J. Lynch and his group at the University of Maryland School of Medicine in Baltimore used this type of recorder to measure blood pressure changes in patients involved in a clinical interview. You might expect your pressure to rise if you're telling the doctor about some painful or disturbing event in your past, or about particular problems in the present.

Surprisingly, Lynch's team found blood pressures increasing even when patients started to answer the simple, unloaded question, 'Tell me about your work.' Hypertensives showed greater increases than normotensives, and patients with the highest resting blood pressures had the highest rises. Some showed a pressure increase of well over a third within half a minute of starting to talk. It fell again just as quickly when they'd finished, and diuretics or even beta-blockers didn't seem to stop it.

Intrigued by these findings the Baltimore group looked at some five hundred subjects aged between three and seventy-five. Nine out of every ten showed a blood pressure rise on speaking or even on reading aloud. And if they were asked to read as fast as possible the rise was greater than when they were reading at their normal, personal tempo. This was true even for young, fit, well-educated volunteers from the hospital staff, much of whose day was spent talking to people. So talking fast and talking loud, two ways that you can tell a Type A even when he's in the next room, may cause some of the blood pressure surges that are the overdriver's trademark.

The Baltimore group recognized the problem. They are currently trying to tackle this talking-induced arousal, by giving volunteers biofeedback of their heart rates and blood pressure responses during the interviews. They hope that the patients will learn to bring them under control. Perhaps eventually, like Bernard Engel and the other Baltimore research team with their home blood pressure monitoring,

Lynch's patients might also be able to learn 'the sense of the biofeedback response'. But however it's done, controlling the Type A's speech patterns ought to be part of the treatment package.

When it comes to competitive drive and impatience, the need to change is also crystal clear. You will remember that Karen Matthews and her colleagues analysed the replies to the structured interview made by sixty-two men in the Western Collaborative Group Study who later went on to show signs of coronary heart disease. By comparing their replies with answers from a group of men in the same study who remained free of CHD, Matthews' team concluded that competitive drive and impatience were the primary Type A risks.

On sub-dividing competitive drive, they found that enjoying competition at work, and showing a high drive level and an easily aroused hostility were especially risky features. So too were having a vigorous answering style and an explosive delivery. Lynch's results, obtained some years later, might explain this part of the risk. You will remember too that Dembroski found competition and hostility to be the hallmarks of those Type As who showed exaggerated responses, whatever the provocation. As to impatience, Matthews found that irritation at waiting in queues and always being punctual for appointments distinguished those men who developed CHD from those who didn't.

It's when we come to *treating* competitive drive and impatience that the problems really begin. Some therapists have tried to teach sufferers to develop a more realistic expectation of their own performance and so lower their competitive demands. They have also tried to teach them better scheduling of their time, to reduce their impatience. Back in 1974, Friedman and Rosenman were recommending that those of us, from salesmen to physicians, who meet a lot of people in our work, shouldn't plan all our day's appointments back-to-back. If you do, you'll inevitably fall behind. And the feeling that you're keeping the *next* client waiting will make you rushed and irritable with the one you're talking to. You'll know and, however hard you try to hide it, he'll know that you're pushed. Robert Eliot suggests that a harried physician should schedule a non-existent patient, some completely fictitious woman, into one of the day's treatment slots. By doing so he gets a chance to calm down, to reflect and to catch up with himself. Eliot explained this to one physician whose chronic impatience shone through his reply – 'What do I do if she doesn't show up?'

Controlling anger is even harder than dealing with time-urgency. Dr Raymond W. Novaco of the University of California at Irvine once made an analysis of the functions that anger serves. They're not all bad, if you have to survive in a constantly hassling world. It's true that anger disrupts whatever you're trying to do, since you can't work properly or even think straight if you're furious. But it also stops you from feeling helpless, and it advertises to the world your sense of potency, expressiveness and determination. As Novaco says: 'It is less distressing to be angry than anxious.' The angry man is saying to anyone who gets in his way, 'There's nothing wrong with me. It's you that's got the problem.'

How do you deal with such an ingrained, self-sustaining attitude? Novaco is a specialist in 'anger management' – a type of therapy designed first of all to give the client some insight into his anger problem. It seems difficult to believe that people whose anger erupts a dozen times a day may hardly notice it. Only when they are asked to keep a diary and note all their angry episodes (justified or not) in the course of a week do many of them even start to appreciate the problem that they're living with.

The next stage is to teach them that an event itself never made anyone angry. It's the way that we see the event, the construction that each of us puts on it, that arouses our anger. It's not having to hit the brake when a car pulls out in front of you that makes you angry on the highway. It's the belief that no one in the world has the right to slow you down that way. It's not the fact that the meal takes an extra five minutes to get to your table that makes you angry in a restaurant. It's the belief that the waiter doesn't think you're important enough to hurry for.

Novaco has produced an inventory of some eighty different situations that are likely to provoke our anger. They range from being served with cold food to being physically assaulted. And all of us can construct our own. Anger management involves confronting each of these situations in your imagination while at the same time defusing the scene by allowing your body to relax completely. Each scene is further defused by repeating to yourself a reasonable, rational self-statement that reflects the situation as it really is, not as you would instantly respond to it. In your car, instead of 'Jesus, what a schmuck' it might be 'That guy's a careless driver, but my brakes and reflexes are good and no harm's been done'. In the restaurant, instead of 'Who does this surly bastard think he's dealing with?' it might be 'I'm in no great hurry, and it's more convenient for me to wait for this meal than to go somewhere else. But I simply shan't come here again.' After enough rehearsal the responses are tried out in real life. When an anger-arousing situation comes along the relaxation can be cued by your breathing and the self-statements keep you rational. The whole object is to remain *task oriented*. Don't let the anger disrupt what you're doing. Don't let it turn your mind to some massive but futile concern with the injustice of the world. What anger management gives above all is a sense of personal control in the handling of provocation.

The crucial importance of reducing angry reactions by whatever means is underlined by a series of findings from the

Department of Psychology at Yale. Dr Gary Schwartz and his associates were interested in what happens to your heart rate and blood pressure when you go through different emotional states. To find out, they had thirty-two college students act out as vividly as possible for themselves the feelings and physical sensations that go with fear, anger and sadness. They did so first while sitting down, then again while exercising on a pair of steps. And at the end of each stage their cardiovascular reactions were measured.

Without doubt anger produced the greatest activation of their cardiovascular systems. While sitting and imagining being angry, the volunteers' diastolic blood pressures rose higher than in any of the other moods. Such a change probably means a constriction of the arteries supplying the body's major muscle groups. It is just the opposite of what happens in exercise where the muscles get an increased blood supply. Schwartz suggests that it may have been a defence for our ancestors against bleeding to death from the injuries sustained in fighting. For us, however, this anger-induced hypertension is anything but protective. It may spell damage both to the coronary arteries and to those supplying the brain. What do we say to the purple-faced man with bulging eyes who's speechless with rage? 'Don't burst a blood vessel.'

During normal exercise, your heart rate and systolic pressure both increase, but when they were exercising during anger, the volunteers' heart rates went up twice as much as normal and their systolic pressures were slow to come down, again creating an added risk of arterial damage, and perhaps of fatal arrhythmias as well. Schwartz endorses the point that I have made already – Type A running may be very different from Type B. He also makes another suggestion that fits in well with Novaco's treatment plan. Whilst relaxation has generally been used in the treatment of anxiety, it may be very valuable in controlling anger reactions as well. No other mood gives greater arousal, and certainly no other mood is in such need of control.

So these are some of the interventions that any programme of behavioural change for overdrivers has to go for – altering speech styles, competitive hostility and outright anger. Different programmes have dealt with different features. None except Friedman's has tried to change them all.

Let's look and see what different counselling groups have actually achieved. In Nebraska, Professor Eliot said that he was more interested in treating hot responders than changing Type A. 'How serious is the type A behavioral pattern?' he asks. 'Must we brainwash all type As until they are modified to more placid Bs? We need to be more selective.' He believes that at least a third and maybe as many as half the American population are hot responders, and that the likelihood of having a second infarction within, say, two years is predicted by whether you are or not. The prediction he claims is independent of whether you're a Type A or B.

But despite these distinctions Eliot still says that the 'most likely candidate for physiological overreactivity – a potential hot reactor' is someone who shows hostility, impatience and individual competitiveness, which he agrees are 'three pre-eminent factors in . . . type A behavior'. So although 'type A behavior is only one piece of the "coronary-prone pie"', what he's actually doing is looking for ways of changing Type A rather than trying to cool the hot responses themselves. Indeed, his only *direct* treatment for hot reactors seems to be use of drugs, particularly beta-blockers. But even he admits that when patients are challenged to do mental tasks like arithmetic, their cardiovascular systems often override the drug effects. Their hot responses simply break through.

The University of Nebraska offered a comprehensive Stress, Health and Physical Evaluation (SHAPE) programme to assess your general health and fitness and to determine whether you were a hot responder. If you were, you might be invited 'to work with a stress therapist, a behavioral consultant, a nutritional expert, an exercise physiologist or another SHAPE professional, best suited to deal with [your] individual needs'. Sessions with the behavioral consultant were aimed at teaching 'behavioural techniques for self mastery'. Eliot talked of changing your perceptions, and setting realistic goals for yourself. He observed how 'our studies show it is desirable to talk to yourself pleasantly'.

Where many specialists would take issue with him is in his suggestion that you should 'assume you have just six months to live. Decide what you really like to do, want to do, and feel you have to do in that limited time. You'll quickly find you have been dealing with a host of unnecessary, unful-filling activities.' This advice is prompted no doubt by Eliot's memories of his own heart attack at the age of forty-four. It comes closer than he might admit to Friedman and Rosen-man's suggestion that we should cultivate the things worth being rather than the things worth having. And like them, he leaves himself open to those who ask, quite reasonably, what would happen if everybody decided to live like that?

Again, the advice that Eliot gives to women who are looking for a self-satisfying identity is 'It's OK to be whatever is OK with you'. But is it? Critics aren't slow to ask what effect this now quaintly dated philosophy with its echoes of Woodstock might have on the way that people live together. Better perhaps to set more modest goals for controlling overdrive, at least to start with. Certainly that is the way the research has developed. Early attempts to change Type A depended on altering one factor or another, and seeing what happened. Only later did therapy develop a more multi-faceted approach.

Perhaps the first of these modest attempts at change dates from 1975, and was devised by Professor Richard M. Suinn of the State University of Colorado at Fort Collins. Suinn's main interest was in the treatment of anxiety. You will recall that following the lead set by Professor Wolpe many psychologists have used (and still use) 'desensitization' for the treatment of phobias. The patient is progressively exposed (first in imagination, then in reality) to the situation that makes him anxious, while at the same time practising relaxation so as to make the graded exposure more tolerable. According to Suinn, the problem with this approach is that you can deal with only one phobia at a time. Getting over a fear of spiders does nothing for your fear of being trapped in a lift.

He therefore decided to concentrate on the physical sensations that we experience when we're exposed to any situation that generates anxiety – maybe your hands clench, your neck muscles tighten or your stomach starts to churn. He believed that controlling these physical reactions would be equivalent to controlling the anxiety itself. So you didn't need a separate treatment for every anxiety source. One technique would do to treat the symptoms, whatever it was out there that was causing them.

The therapy consists first of drawing up a set of detailed descriptions of the sort of situations that make the patient feel anxious. These are contrasted with another set of imaginary scenes in which he or she feels relaxed. During treatment sessions patients first imagine an anxiety-provoking scene. Then they relax and switch in imagination to a pleasant one. The effect is to turn the anxiety off again. This is repeated many times so the patient comes to recognize the body cues associated with anxiety. By relaxing them away as soon as they occur, patients learn to prevent the anxiety attack itself. From the therapist's office they take what they have learned out into the real world and use their cue-induced relaxation to deal with the onset of any anxiety the moment their bodies start to feel uneasy.

I have said several times that anxiety isn't the overdriver's main problem. But I've also said, and this is Suinn's rationale, that the Type A constantly puts himself into provoking situations – occasions that make him over-react. Being able to recognize and deal with the way his body responds under provocation would be enormously valuable to him, and we have already seen several attempts to get him to do just that, by switching on the sense of relaxation or the sense of feedback.

What Suinn did initially was to instruct a group of ten coronary patients in the imagery and relaxation technique. The emphasis was on a short form of therapy. Patients learned deep muscle relaxation in less than an hour, and the whole programme was completed with only five hours of patient contact. He stressed that they were acquiring behavioural skills, methods of coping. The technique was simply a procedure to be learned. It didn't depend on psychotherapy or on self-analysis to gain a greater understanding of their underlying conflicts or emotions.

He used a fall in cholesterol as a measure of improved coping in these coronary patients, and he found an average fall of 7 per cent as a result of practising the therapy. A group of similar patients who weren't taught the method showed no change. Encouraged by this he repeated it on a second group of seventeen post-coronaries with much the same result.

Of course, cholesterol falls are interesting as a measure of distress, but they don't tell you much about Type A. Infarction patients don't tell you a great deal about healthy Type As either. So Suinn, together with Dr Larry J. Bloom, went on to treat seven volunteers who answered a newspaper advertisement for normal Type A subjects. They included a sales manager, an executive secretary and a mathematician. They went through six sessions of anxiety management training, with particular emphasis on the control of their time-urgency. Before and after the three-week programme their Type A was measured with the JAS, and so were their anxiety, blood pressure and cholesterol levels.

Unfortunately, the results weren't nearly as promising

with these healthy volunteers as in the more highly motivated coronary population. The effect of treatment was to reduce their scores on the Hard-Driving scale of the JAS questionnaire, but their overall Type A scores didn't shift significantly. Anxiety levels after treatment were lower than in a group who hadn't been treated, but blood pressures showed no significant change and cholesterol actually went up.

So anxiety management may be good for anxiety, but treating the overdriver needs something else. Perhaps that something is a 'cognitive therapy' – a way of getting people to change their unreasonable beliefs about themselves and their world, and to substitute instead a set of more rational opinions about how things really are.

Most of us carry around a set of deep-seated misconceptions about how things ought to be. Common ones include: 'Everyone must love me; everything I do must be perfect; I must always succeed at everything.' Of course we don't entertain them in this transparent form. We disguise them, even to ourselves, and we would vigorously deny thinking them at all if someone accused us of it. But Dr Albert Ellis, a New York psychologist, became famous in the 1960s for suggesting that such ideas should not simply be suppressed. Instead, they should be positively rejected and more reasonable and liveable expectations should be substituted for them. So, for example, 'Everyone must love me' should become 'It's nice, though not essential for an adult to be loved by other people. But it's better to stand on your own feet than depend on others.'

You will recognize many of these irrational beliefs in the make-up of the Type A1, and Mary A. Jenni and Dr Janet P. Wollersheim of the University of Montana were among the first to see what effect changing irrational beliefs might have on the intensity of Type A behaviour. As part of Mary Jenni's doctoral project they recruited sixteen Type A1s and twenty-six A2s, most of them in positions of 'initiative and responsibility', into a therapy programme involving six once-weekly sessions, each lasting for ninety minutes.

The volunteers were split into two groups and half were given cognitive therapy. They were taught how to recognize the bodily feelings that meant they were getting tense, and then to look at their beliefs about the sources of the tension to decide whether they were reasonable or not. If not, they learned how to make more reasonable statements to themselves. For example, much of the tension, disappointment and anger felt by these Type As resulted from them constantly competing, not with other people, but with their own impossibly high standards. The therapist showed them that what they were saying, in effect, was 'I must always be perfect' – a quite unliveable expectation. In its place was substituted a much more obtainable goal like 'I will do my best, but if it's less than perfect I won't get upset'. The other half of the volunteer group were given anxiety management training using audio tapes produced by Richard Suinn, and the two approaches were compared.

Both procedures reduced the volunteers' anxiety and the way that it showed itself in symptoms like muscle tension, chest pain, becoming less effective and 'getting nasty'. Only the cognitive approach produced any change in Type A behaviour, and even that was small. It was limited to the A1s and it was measured only by the volunteers' own assessment of how they had changed.

Nonetheless, as the researchers remarked, any success was welcome, particularly as they hadn't asked volunteers to slow down at all. Indeed, the clients' high drives for success had actually been used as a motivating factor. Several of them had to be specifically assured that entering the programme would not make them less achieving. They were told that, on the contrary, they could *increase* their competence by learning to relax their tensions.

That particular sales pitch – 'reduce your Type A to increase your effectiveness' – has a lot to be said for it. It is an offer that the overdriver can hardly refuse. And it has been used to great effect by a research group in Montreal.

'Motivating people to participate in a Type A intervention program involves persuading individuals to change a deeply rooted, gratifying and socially approved lifestyle for the sake of health benefits that are still very uncertain.' If this statement from Ethel Roskies, Professor of Psychology at the University of Montreal, sounds pessimistic, it arises from the frustrating experience of trying to bring such changes about. Time and again the volunteers in her counselling sessions found reasons why they should hang on to their Type A habits. Wasn't it true that you had to blow off steam now and again? If you bottled it all up wouldn't that affect your health? And wouldn't controlling your anger produce a sort of emotional flatness that would make it difficult for you to respond to any aspect of your life, good or bad?

Roskies faced this question of how to change a highly valued lifestyle head on. She admits that in the last analysis Type As might need a complete overhaul of their personal philosophy of life before they can really change – the sort of reorientation that Friedman and Rosenman were describing a decade ago. But she believes that going in that direction might itself produce a host of problems, for the sufferer himself no less than for his family and for the organization that employs him. At a more practical level, she points out that few Type As, if any, are likely to volunteer for any programme aimed at producing such a drastic shift in their orientation. Only if less radical programmes fail does she feel we are justified in trying to produce such fundamental changes in the Type A's whole attitude to his world.

Her own approach is based upon the ideas of David Glass and Karen Matthews, both of whom suggested that the Type A is a person who has become obsessed with the need to control his environment. Any threat to this sense of mastery produces a burst of furious activity in an attempt to get back on top. It produces frequent bouts of anger as well, though Roskies asks an intriguing question. Is the Type A's anger more often and more easily provoked than the Type B's, or when the Type A gets aroused, is he simply more likely to *label* his arousal as anger? In other words, will he tend to feel angry in almost any situation where he has to make an effort? If so, he really is locked in, because effort (and competitive effort at that) is the mainspring of his life.

Either way, if his need for control is the key, then there are several ways he might be helped. Roskies rejects the idea of trying to change his working environment so that there are fewer challenges in it. At present it just isn't practical to think of altering working practices, at least until we can be more sure of the results. That was the whole problem with the Swedish findings on effort and distress. Though jobs can be redesigned to separate the two, few corporations are interested in doing so at a time when demand and output are falling.

That leaves us with two options. Either we can try to change the Type A's perceptions, so that he feels fewer situations as threatening. In that way we reduce his need to be constantly mobilizing to meet the challenge. Or we can teach him more effective ways of coping with challenge when it does come along, and so reduce the intensity of his reaction to it. That is, we can teach him coping skills to weave into the fabric of his daily life. Roskies' team tried both.

The way they recruited their first group of subjects was an object lesson in tapping into Type A attitudes. They wanted thirty Type A1s aged between thirty-five and fifty-nine. They had to be free from coronary disease and not on any major medication. They had to be in professional or executive jobs, earning at least $25,000 when they entered the study in 1977. They had to be prepared to attend at least twelve out of fourteen weekly ninety-minute therapy sessions and they had to pay a deposit of $100 which was returned only if their attendance was satisfactory.

Finding enough men who satisfied these criteria might seem almost impossible, and certainly a month of talking to corporate executives and their physicians produced few results. So the research team went public. They produced a newspaper article and radio interview in which the treatment programme was explained. Rather than concentrating on Type A as a coronary risk factor, it was described as an inefficient way of behaving, like running your engine at full speed the whole time. The promise of the treatment programme was that without altering the volunteers' need or capacity to get things done, he would learn how to 'accomplish more with less strain'. But positions on the course were limited. They could only take thirty.

They got one hundred and fifty phone calls in three days. They had pitched the message just right to appeal to the Type A's competitive instincts, and indeed many of the volunteers complimented the team on the businesslike way they had set the whole thing up.

Twenty-five Type A1s were selected and completed the course. Following the system we have seen so often, they were divided into two groups. For thirteen of them the intention was to change their perceptions of possible threats and hence reduce the need that they felt to be always in control. For this they received treatment from psychotherapists who suggested to them that their urge to achieve sprang from their childhood, where they had an aggressive, demanding mother and a passive or absent father. They were still in effect striving to obtain their mother's love. The purpose of the therapy was to make them realize how their current behaviour was no more than 'the replaying of an out-dated family script'. This psychoanalytic approach was administered by therapists who genuinely believed in its potential value for treating Type As. It wasn't some dummy method like Jonathan Smith's periodic somatic inactivity, laid on just to produce a comparison group. For the therapists themselves it was for real.

The other group of Type As were taught progressive relaxation. First they went through a full fifteen-minute version, then after four weeks it was reduced to five minutes. Four weeks later they were taught to relax on cue, particular cues being, for example, every time the phone rang or every time they found themselves in a disagreement at work. Even at the start of the treatment most of the men thought that they were fairly relaxed already. One of the major tasks was to get them to monitor their levels of tension and discover just how up-tight they actually were. Eventually they built a regular check into their daily routine, scanning their muscles for tension while they were shaving, driving and so on.

And did the psychotherapy or the relaxation have any effect on their Type A behaviour? Roskies claims that neither the structured interview nor the JAS are sensitive enough to be able to do proper before-and-after comparisons, so the question can't be answered directly. However, the subjects' sense of time pressure had decreased by the end of the course as a result of relaxation. So too had their cholesterol levels and systolic blood pressures. Unfortunately for the study (though not for the patients) similar falls occurred in the psychotherapy group as well.

Some specialists will see these results as confirming that it doesn't actually matter what you do to patients to produce psychological changes. All that matters is the amount of time you spend with them. Certainly the psychotherapy results are striking. Six months after the study had finished the men in this group still continued to show a slightly greater systolic fall than had the normotensive men in Wilmington who practised the twelve weeks of Benson's relaxation response.

But more interesting than resting blood pressure levels are the pressure responses that occur as a result of challenge. It was that reactivity that Roskies and her group set out to measure in a second investigation involving sixty-six middle managers. It would be nice to report that they sewed the subject up, and that they showed similar reactivity results to Chandra Patel, but on a bigger scale. Unfortunately, they didn't. Perhaps because of the problems that they found with the measurements and the equipment, they haven't so far managed to show any change in blood pressure reactivity as a result of any Type A intervention programme. But that's not to say that they won't. In 1981 Roskies declared that: 'Because we believe that reducing the frequency, intensity and duration of sympathetic arousal is, in the current state of our knowledge, the most viable therapeutic target for Type A intervention . . . we shall continue to pursue this goal.' Despite the failure of their second study, their approach itself is well worth looking at.

The executives in Roskies' first trial noticed that although relaxation had beneficial effects on muscle tension, their problems also took other forms. They had periods of obsessive worrying and times when their thoughts went racing – situations that relaxation could do little about. What they needed was some way of coping – indeed more than one way – to deal with the variety of problems that they faced.

So in addition to relaxation on cue, for example, whenever they caught sight of the red stars they had stuck around the office, they were also taught that their feelings resulted from how they saw a situation, not from the situation itself. Those irrational beliefs which lead to negative feelings should simply be thrown away. In their place, they should put more reasonable self-statements. Familiar? Yes, it's the change of thinking pioneered by Albert Ellis and used for Type As by Mary Jenni and (as we shall see) by Friedman's group.

In Roskies' second study, volunteers were asked to record

a couple of upsetting incidents, as and when they actually happened. Then later they 'replayed' the experiences, and examined their reactions to them, looking for ways that they would have thought, and hence acted, differently. They also went through imaginary situations, deliberately modifying their reactions and noticing the statements that had helped to defuse the problem. Finally, they were taught to handle real events as they occurred and to try, as Roskies puts it, 'to shift their feelings into a lower key . . . irritation, annoyance, frustration, disappointment . . . were suggested as more rational responses than fury'. When combined with relaxation, this type of rethinking was particularly effective for keeping arousal levels down.

Sometimes the Type A's sense of time-urgency, quite apart from his anger, can get so bad that it stops him momentarily from doing anything at all. Most of us have felt the paralysis that comes from suddenly realizing that we can't possibly get through it all today, but knowing at the same time that we've got to. Part of the answer lies in planning your time better, in deciding what (if anything) is urgent, and then dealing with that first. If everything has a number one priority, nothing gets done at all. Part of the answer also lies in refusing to get overwhelmed by the deadlines other people would lay on you – 'Do you want it tomorrow or do you want it right?'

But even if you are used to managing your time well, it's often impossible to stay completely cool when the pressure's really on. The trick is to keep functioning, pressured or not, instead of going to pieces. And that again has to do with being able to relax and generate the right sort of statements for yourself. Instead of 'I'm never going to get through all this' try 'I've got through workloads like this before. It may take an extra day, but I'm not going to get upset about that.' Instead of 'If the costings come through in today's mail I'll have to drop everything to read them' try 'If they arrive I'll file them and deal with them when I can'. Instead of 'My secretary looks at me like I'm burnt out' try 'Does she pay my salary or do I pay hers?'

After attending a dozen sessions to learn these principles, many of the middle managers in Roskies' second group felt an increased sense of life satisfaction. They especially felt that they were more in control than they had been before they enrolled. In that respect, and in the fact that they joined and stuck at the programme at all, it was a success. But since it didn't show any change in heart rate or blood pressure reactivity on or off the job, and since that was the specific goal that the researchers had set themselves, then it had to be seen as a failure. The question which the Montreal team are engaged in solving now, is whether the failure really was due to technical problems. Or was the lack of any major change perhaps the inevitable consequence of using a programme that was only brief, to produce changes that were only superficial? Maybe the only way to save the overdriver from himself really is to rebuild his whole philosophy of life after all – just what the Recurrent Coronary Prevention Project aimed to do.

This project originated from a meeting that Meyer Friedman had with Carl E. Thoresen, who was Professor of Education at Stanford University and a specialist in the newly emerging subject of behaviour therapy. At just the same time that Friedman and Rosenman were publishing *Type A Behavior and Your Heart* with its suggested formulae for changing yourself, Thoresen, together with Michael J. Mahoney of Pennsylvania State University, had produced *Behavioral Self-Control*. This was a short general summary of some of the ways in which our behaviour can be altered for our benefit. It looked at progress during the previous decade or so in the psychological treatment that came to be known as behaviour therapy. We've had glimpses of it already – Ellis's rational self-statements, Suinn's anxiety treatment, Novaco's anger management. It was natural then that Friedman, who knew little about psychology, and Thoresen, who at the time knew equally little about cardiology, should attempt to combine their expertise to set up a programme of behavioural change for Type As. Others also became involved, such as Dr James T. Gill, another principal investigator.

Recruiting patients into the trial began in 1977 and occupied the greater part of 1978. From the outset they decided to study individuals who had already suffered at least one infarction. The reason was simple. These post-MI patients were six times more likely to have another infarction than people who hadn't had a heart attack. So the question 'Will changing Type A behaviour lower the infarction rate?' could be answered much more quickly for that group than for healthy Type As. They hoped to get an answer within five years.

Assembling the thousand patients or so that they needed was a major undertaking. The advertisement in *Time* was only a small part of it. In addition they enlisted the help of cardiologists and internists, corporate and union executives, local newspaper editors and radio and TV directors to get across the message that the trial was looking for volunteers. The subjects they got, as in the Western Collaborative Group Study, were mostly middle-class corporate employees. Their average age was fifty-four. Nine out of ten were men. While all had suffered at least one heart attack, several had had two infarctions or more.

Obviously, all post-coronary patients need the regular care of their personal physician. They also need to know about and to benefit from the latest findings in coronary research. So as well as their usual physician's care, all of the actively treated patients involved in the RCPP also received expert advice and counselling from a cardiologist. For some, that was the only advice they did receive. In addition, a second group got special counselling on how to change their Type A behaviour. And a third, who were examined only at the beginning and end of the study, acted as a comparison, to see what happened to post-MI patients attending their own physician but not receiving counselling of any kind.

Once the volunteers had been accepted for the trial and had, for their part, accepted to participate in it, they were allocated to one of the groups. Roughly three hundred were selected for counselling by the cardiologist alone. Twice as many were put into the behaviour change group, because the investigators expected far more of them to find commitment to changing their lives so great that they would leave the study before it was finished. In the event, this prediction proved to be wrong. Individuals did 'drop out', but they dropped out of the two groups at the same rate. Type A counselling was no more (or less) exacting than sessions with the cardiologist.

But how could any treatment be provided for such large numbers? Obviously, not on a one-to-one basis. Instead, it was decided to divide the volunteers up into groups of ten or twelve, and all treatment advice would be given on this small group basis. With so many patients it was necessary to form over eighty groups, each with their individual group leader, either a cardiologist, a psychologist or psychiatrist concerned with behavioural change. After the first three months of twice-weekly then monthly meetings, the cardiologist-led groups met once every two months. Each meeting lasted for an hour and a half. Groups led by the psychologists or psychiatrists met monthly. They did so because in addition to their behavioural change, these patients had to get the same amount of cardiological advice as well. In retrospect, this small group format, each with its own group leader, proved to be an excellent way of getting the message across.

We have seen that the all-important questions that the RCPP was designed to address were firstly whether Type A could be altered and secondly, if it could, what effect the change would have on the pattern of reinfarction. To answer the first, it was essential to be able to measure Type A, and more especially to be able to measure Type A changes over time. And that's not easy. You may remember Ethel Roskies deciding that it wasn't even possible, and choosing to look at serum cholesterol or reactivity instead.

The RCPP approached the problem of measuring change in two ways. First, when the participants entered the study and again at the end of each year of treatment, they answered a questionnaire about the intensity of their time-urgency and hostility, as they felt it both at work and at home. It contained questions like 'How often do you feel compelled in conversing with people *to get your thoughts across quickly* because you feel they may not have enough time to listen to you?' and 'How annoyed or irritated do you become with the excess of repetitive, sometimes nonsensical details associated with your job?' Respondents scored their answers on a scale from 1 to 5 and their total scores on these nearly ninety questions gave a measure of their behaviour and, more importantly, of how it might change from year to year. Their spouse, and a close friend, also answered similar questionnaires about them, as a cross-check on how accurate the subject's own answers were.

But with all that we have said about Type A questionnaires like the JAS and the Framingham scale, it's obvious that this one as well can have only a limited value. A more objective measure of how the volunteers had changed was sought by using the Videotaped Structured Interview, or VSI. You will recall that from his experience of what he judged Type As to be really like, after seeing many hundreds of them, Meyer Friedman added a number of behavioural clues to his diagnosis of the Type A pattern. So, in addition to the actual interview answers and the speed and force of the subject's voice while answering (all of which were assessed in the

WCGS) he added features like rapid head nodding, knee jiggling, tongue clicking and the showing of a clenched fist. In the RCPP, subjects went through a structured interview of twenty-eight questions, some concerned with how their lives had changed since their heart attack. Their responses were recorded on video and their various Type A features, both vocal and visual, were given a score which depended on their frequency and intensity. The total was the VSI score, and it was measured both when the subjects entered the trial and at the end of three years of treatment.

It has to be said that some Type A specialists doubt whether many of the visual clues, like sweat on the forehead, a tense facial expression or the presence of black pigmented rings under the eyes are Type A indicators at all. Since they weren't measured in the WCGS we don't know if they're really associated with an increased coronary risk. We will only know that when the RCPP team discovers whether they occur more often among the reinfarction victims – a project that is now well in hand.

In the meantime, however, there seems little doubt that three years of behavioural counselling produced a real fall in the intensity of the Type A pattern. The average scores on the patients' own questionnaires, and on those filled in by their spouse and friend, all fell during the course of the study. Their VSI scores fell too. We have seen many times that simply being involved in this type of study, even if you are not in the 'active' group, often brings some benefit (remember the Australian blood pressure trial?). So it was not surprising that the patients who just got cardiological counselling also showed some Type A change. But the shift was greater among the behaviour change groups than among those led by the cardiologists. By the end of the second year, about half of the Type A counselled patients had shown some decrease in the intensity of their behaviour. For the cardiologist-led groups, the improvement was only a third.

Interestingly enough, most of the changes that did occur seemed to do so during the first year. Those who were going to get the message got it early. A look at those who dropped out is equally revealing. They seemed to be individuals high on hostility but low on social support, exactly those who would have benefited most from persisting. Or would they? Because the bottom line of all of this is not really whether the questionnaires or interview ratings changed. The whole point was to see whether the rate of reinfarction was reduced by behavioural change more than by cardiological counselling alone, or indeed more than by doing nothing beyond what your own physician recommends.

When the study was terminated, the reinfarction rate in the behaviour change group was about half that found in the cardiologist and control groups combined. Even biasing the figures against success, by including those patients who dropped out and so denied themselves therapy while continuing to carry the same coronary risk, the behaviour change group still had the lowest reinfarction rate. We can look at the figures another way, and separate those subjects who showed a behavioural change in the first year from those who didn't. The ones who got the message and got it early had only a quarter as much reinfarction as those showing no change in behaviour at the end of the study. So the answer was clear.

All of these differences were in *non-fatal* recurrences. The death rates showed a similar trend but were not so clear-cut. Why? Probably because in such an intensive study, where patients and their relatives were acutely sensitive to the signals of any impending attack, the family was extremely good at getting the patient to hospital at the first hint of trouble. They had perhaps learned the hard way to avoid the denial and delays that can prove fatal. Instead they were geared up for quick action to save his life.

Even so, some died. Whenever possible, after each attack,

the research team tried to establish from the sufferer if he survived, or from his relatives if not, exactly what he was doing when the attack came on. In two cases out of three it was just what he had been warned about time and again – quarrelling with business associates or members of the family, allowing himself to get exhausted or over-excited, or eating a heavy fat meal.

But it's no good saying 'If only they'd listened, the trial results would have been better', because what was on trial was whether this type of counselling with its small group format could make patients listen and learn and remember. And it did. Even with its problem patients the RCPP did better than any other Type A intervention. What's the magic formula that the counsellors used? Their approach is what specialists call 'eclectic'. That means you take a bit of everything from everywhere.

Not that it's haphazard. On the contrary. The treatment is based firmly on the idea that Type A is an over-learned behaviour, an inappropriate way of solving problems that has become deeply internalized. We've seen why many times. In the short term, it works. The RCPP belief was that it can be *unlearned* again, but for that to happen more appropriate behaviours have to be put in its place. Since Type A colours not only our actions but also the way that we think and feel about everything, including our relationships with other people, the therapy has to influence all of these areas – hence the eclectic approach to change first the outward behaviour, then the attitudes behind it.

So let's look at a few of the skills that Type As can be taught. First, they can learn muscle relaxation, the basic exercise that makes it easier for most people to start dealing with their anxieties or their anger. Many Type As actually resist it at first. They find the inactivity positively unpleasant, at least until they have learned some form of mental relaxation as well, perhaps by focusing on their breathing, with an exercise like Chandra Patel's.

However good you are at relaxing and finding calm 'inside', you make life difficult for yourself if you allow your surroundings to keep throwing unnecessary challenges at you. Most of us have jobs that call for effort and generate some distress. But there are usually ways of reducing both, and it's only common sense to do so. The RCPP encouraged its volunteers to allocate priorities in their daily workload; to schedule time in the day to *allow* for things going wrong; not to take on additional jobs without being able to offload some of those already on their desk; and perhaps above all to schedule some time in the day *for themselves*. Relationships with work colleagues can be a particular source of strain and the Project used the Novaco Anger Scale to let volunteers assess for themselves, *in advance*, those situations most likely to make them explode. They could then work *in advance* on facing them more rationally.

It's not just at work that problems like these surface. The MI patients were also encouraged to look at the problems that arose at home, with their wives and children, and to take time out to deal with them. At the very least they were recommended to spend half an hour a month in a 'discuss/ review' session with their wives, where areas of conflict could be resolved. It was even suggested that they take more time to be friendly with their neighbours.

As well as reorganizing their environment, a major part of the RCPP training was in learning to avoid the exaggerated arousal to which they had been prone for years. The first step was to be able to see it, and much time in the early sessions was concerned with self-observation and self-assessment. In this, the other group members provided an invaluable mirror for each individual to see himself as the others saw him. Since they all had the same problem, their observations of each other were razor-sharp. It was the group leader's task to show how the observers themselves were just as guilty.

Having gained a little, painful insight into how easily they erupted, a major goal of treatment was to teach them how to start avoiding it. The first thing to change was their 'self-talk' – the incessant monologue that goes on all the time in all our heads. Instead of a stream of thinking about the constant challenge, the blind unfairness and the relentless struggle in their lives, they were taught how their self-talk could be more calm and reassuring. They learned how to take the arousal out of many situations, as a result of what they told themselves.

But talking to yourself isn't enough. You also have to act, and before anyone can act, they have to rehearse. So the volunteer patients actually rehearsed new ways of acting, like talking more slowly and interrupting less, moving more slowly and gesturing less, and letting the tension go out of their faces. To help with this last exercise they were encouraged to look deeply into the faces of other people, something they'd never done before. They started to see the difference between those who were chronically stressed and aroused and those who were more calm and tranquil, and started to practise being more like the second. Having practised on their own and in the group they took this collection of acts, this 'behavioural rehearsal', into use in their everyday lives. To explain how anything so apparently artificial can eventually become a part of you, Friedman is fond of quoting Hamlet's advice to his mother: 'Assume a virtue, if you have it not.' In other words: 'If you act like it, you'll get like it.'

Finally, the RCPP volunteers learned to examine their own underlying beliefs and values in a searching and critical way. This is something that all of us find difficult, but the small group format gave them support. They looked at how their perceptions of the world influenced the way that they acted, often quite unreasonably. They considered their self-image and asked themselves whether it really mirrored their range of abilities and limitations. They also discussed their hostility, their distrust, their suspicion and their all-too-ready criticism of others. We have looked at the Type A's distorted core beliefs already, and these patients were invited to do the same.

That, in essence, is the RCPP treatment package. Most of the components we've seen before. But here, for the first time, they were mixed and matched for a very specific purpose – to prevent the sort of behaviour that leads to reinfarction. As I've described it, the treatment might seem rather intense, but the subjects didn't have it thrust on them all at once, and the atmosphere in the groups that I attended was anything but heavy. Certainly, all the participants realized that they were dealing with a life-or-death issue, but most of them approached it with good humour. And their sense of humour was constantly encouraged by the group leaders as a way of defusing their personal and their mutual hostilities.

In the early days, the leaders often had such hostility turned on them. Every assumption, every recommendation was questioned by patients who thought (and said) that twenty minutes of relaxation every day was ridiculous, or that driving in the slow lane couldn't possibly do anything for their heart condition. Both the leader's replies and (even more so) the way that he or she reacted to such a critical deluge provided an invaluable model for the group. For the first time in years, many of them saw someone they respected acting in a patient and accepted manner under provocation. If the leaders could do it, the members could do it as well.

But how were the groups actually conducted? What went on for ninety minutes every month? A typical group meeting woud start with a relaxation exercise. Then the members went on to discuss this month's *bomb and fuse*. Since Type As have a keen sense of the dramatic, and since they best remember ideas that are practical, Friedman told them that each one was carrying a bomb around in his chest. The bomb was the liability that they had to live with, the result of having an area of infarcted myocardium probably with blocked coronary arteries as well. It could easily explode, and the explosion might be fatal – either another infarction or a sudden arrhythmic death. But, they were told, a bomb will not explode without a fuse, and the patients needed to know what the fuses were so that they could avoid them. Four of the most important are summarized by Friedman's formula AIAI. They are anger, irritation, aggression and impatience. Other fuses are physical exhaustion, mental exertion and a heavy fat meal. The latter is dangerous not because it puts long-term cholesterol levels up, but because in the short term it apparently leads to clumping or sludging of red blood cells, which makes it more difficult for them to get through narrow blood vessels and to deliver oxygen where it's needed.

At each meeting the group looked at the bomb and its fuses and each man asked himself 'Where did I go wrong this month; where did I risk igniting the fuse?' If anyone in the entire study had died or had a recurrence since the last session his case was reviewed by the whole group. This time they asked 'Where did *he* go wrong?' Often the answer was plain enough, and it served as a dramatic reminder to the others.

After the bomb and fuses, the group went on to discuss its drills. As we have seen time and again, monthly or even weekly group sessions are not enough to change your behaviour in any fundamental way. You have to practise outside, every day in real life. To help them, each patient in the behaviour change group had a *Drill Book* that listed a separate drill to practise for each day of the week. For example, on Wednesdays in January the drill was 'leave watch off'. On Thursdays it was 'walk more slowly' and on Sundays 'practise smiling'. This last one produces some interesting results. Try it yourself. If you're a man, the effect of smiling at women can be very gratifying. Smiling at other men takes more courage. Drills for March included 'seek a long line in a store or bank' (a sure sign you're recovering if you can stand there calmly) and 'linger at table'. For Fridays in August the drill was 'purposely say "maybe I'm wrong"', one of the most difficult and most valuable of them all.

The Drill Book is also full of quotations for you to think about during the week. It's easy enough to be turned off by this sort of Readers' Digest Condensed Wisdom but some of the quotes are worth thinking about for months rather than weeks. For example, what about Lord Chesterfield's 'Whoever is in a hurry shows that the thing he is about to do is too big for him' or Norman Mailer's 'The religion of the rich is the freedom from dread' or F. Scott Fitzgerald's 'There is no second act in American lives'?

After the drills, the groups went on to look at particular problems that any of the members might have had, like containing their anger. If, for example, one of them had his hostility aroused by the rudeness and indifference of a shop assistant, another member of the group might play the part of the assistant, and he and the victim would re-enact the scene for everyone to see. This gave the victim an opportunity to look again at what he actually did so that he could act differently next time. It gave the group members the chance of suggesting alternative ways of behaving, both for him and for themselves, and it gave the 'assistant' the chance to see the whole incident from the real assistant's point of view, which might make him a little more compassionate the next time.

After discussing any new research findings on Type A that might have recently come to light and that they could apply to themselves, and after setting the homework assignments for them to concentrate on until the next session, the group meetings concluded with a prayer. It was a non-sectarian prayer, but a prayer nonetheless, in which the patients admitted that they were there because they needed help, and prayed that friendship and *love* (they weren't afraid of the word) might enrich their lives and the lives of those in their care.

So the final ingredient in the eclectic parcel is a spiritual one. And we shouldn't be too surprised. In conversation, and in his writings, Friedman has often described Type A behaviour as a 'spiritual disease', which could only benefit from a spiritual remedy.

But other specialists disagree, some of them profoundly. First, they object to it being called a disease at all. Type A *leads* to disease, but what makes it so difficult to deal with is the very fact that those who've got it know they're not sick – at least not physically and not yet. As to 'spiritual', other experts wonder if the label is the least bit helpful when it comes to counselling the successful Type A at the height of his career. You might treat men in their sixties with a spiritual programme. There's a very telling line in *Type A Behavior and Your Heart* about how little you need to live well and happily 'Especially as you pass sixty-five . . .' But you don't treat thirty-year-olds that way. Indeed, it is my belief that you don't waste your time trying to treat men of thirty for Type A at all.

12. Saving Your Own Life

I was once in a plane between New York and Chicago, on the way to California to learn how to do the structured interview. My wife had fallen asleep and I was reading a very dense article on Type A, the report of an expert review panel convened specially in 1978 by the National Heart, Lung and Blood Institute 'to determine the efficacy and relevance of this research to the prevention and control of CHD'.

I'd become vaguely aware of a slightly overweight, youngish-looking man on my other side before we took off. Somehow he'd managed to get on the plane before the rest of us and had even got himself a glass of water. He had also refused to fasten his seat belt until we were practically airborne. 'Sometimes,' he told me, 'they keep you on the taxi-way for half an hour.'

The moment I put the report down I was aware of him again. 'Do you mind if I read your paper?' Obviously he'd been glancing over my shoulder. I explained that it was really a heavyweight publication produced by one group of specialists for another, but he was undeterred. He studied it avidly for perhaps fifteen minutes, particularly the last section on Type A intervention. Turning to me he said: 'I'm really very interested in all this. I think some of it might apply to me.' Then he told me the life story of a super-A.

He was thirty-three and over the previous five years he had built up a small marketing consultancy into a $5 million business. As well as getting wealthy he had also gained respect and a reputation. As we met, he was on his way as an invited guest speaker to a business convention. But, he told me, he was suffering from the effects of success. It had all come very quickly, and he wasn't sure how to handle it. He was in analysis to treat his 'anxiety' but he didn't seem the least anxious or neurotic to me. The problem was that he had no criteria of success. Before he started the business he hadn't any clear idea where he wanted to go, and so he had no way of knowing whether he'd arrived. He just kept on acquiring things that he didn't need, almost by habit.

I wondered what drove him to live the life that he did. He said that ever since he was a kid he'd tried to impress people, to make up for the fact that his father had never loved him. And he was still trying. Then, quite out of the blue he confessed to me that some people like him generated aggravation just for the excitement of it. They almost seemed to have a death wish. He had a partner who was constantly creating conflict when there was no reason to do so. He just couldn't seem to live in a more tranquil environment. My friend wondered whether he was subconsciously trying to bring his death closer, to kill himself by working, and so capture everyone's admiration. In short, to gain death with honour.

I explained that he was the classic Type A. I said that if he hadn't told me all this (and I have not embroidered any of it) I couldn't have created a better example of a Type A character. And I told him about the efforts that were being made to help him and people like him. When I got to San Francisco I described my encounter at the group leaders' meeting. They were less impressed with my ready-made archetype than I'd expected. After thinking for a while I realized why. They see men like him all the time.

Well, perhaps not quite like him. Because what impressed me most about the man in the next seat wasn't so much his textbook portrayal of the Type A1 as the fact that, at thirty-three, he was eager to do something about it. Few men of his age are. He was a special case, and there were two features that made him special. First, his rise had been especially rapid. He had focused all the pressures that most men experience over a decade or two, into a space of five years. So his problem was particularly acute. It's no coincidence that Canadian studies found the highest concentration of Type As in the fastest growing companies, where the work force had to make the greatest effort in the shortest time.

But he was special too in having got to the top, or at least high enough to be able to step back and reflect on his situation. Most men of his age aren't able to. They're too busy getting on. The same Canadian investigators found the majority of Type As among the middle management. While three managers out of four were Type A in the survey as a whole, among the most senior executives there was a greater proportion of Bs. Whether they were always Bs who got to the top through their unhurried creativity, or whether they were As who reformed once they reached a position to do so, is one of the great unanswered questions. Either way, the fact remains that even to contemplate change you have to be in a suitable place to contemplate it from.

And you have to have a good reason for wanting to. My friend saw the death wish in his colleague. He didn't want to go the same way. But for most thirty-year-olds the idea of a work-induced heart attack seems extremely remote. The statistics agree. Fatal infarctions in American men between twenty-five and thirty-four run at perhaps one in 20,000. Less than a thousand such deaths occurred in the whole United States in 1976. But go up a decade and the situation starts to change. There were five times as many among men aged thirty-five to forty-four, and twenty times more for men between forty-five and fifty-four. Forty then is perhaps the age to start getting concerned, the age when you can't ignore the statistics any longer.

I say that knowing only too well that by then the overdriver has been damaging his arteries for a decade or two. I say it well aware that 'primary prevention' should start in childhood and that by forty we may have missed the chance to save twenty-five years of atheroma, arrhythmias and clotting platelets.

But have we really missed it? We can hardly blame ourselves for missing a chance that never existed. And for nine overdrivers out of ten, the possibility of changing sooner is simply a non-starter. First he has to get where he's going. I reached this conclusion not only from my personal experience and the experience of my friends (and probably your friends too). I have a more documented reason for believing it as well.

Daniel J. Levinson is Professor of Psychology in the Department of Psychiatry at Yale. In 1966, at the age of forty-six, with a deep personal as well as professional interest in what happens to men in their middle years, he and his colleagues began a series of in-depth interviews with forty American men, writers and manual workers, scientists and executives, aged between twenty-five and forty-five. The object was to trace the course of their adult development. The findings were reported in the research team's book *The Seasons of a Man's Life*.

To summarize very briefly, they discovered that from the age of entering adulthood at about twenty-two, all the men's lives developed through a series of periods and transitions, and that, whatever their jobs, there was a remarkable similarity between what happened in these periods and the ages at which the various men reached them.

For example, the time from twenty-two to twenty-eight (give or take one or two years) was the first part of the 'novice phase'. The primary and overriding task during this period was to make a place for yourself in the adult world. For all four occupations this meant hard work and often a good deal of dedication. Even so, the life situation that they all faced in their late twenties was 'unstable, incomplete and fragmented'.

Between twenty-eight and thirty-four there followed a transition, a feeling that 'this is the time for change', often a time of crisis, when the men seemed to be in 'imminent danger of chaos, dissolution, loss of the future'. But the transition came to an end after about five years and there followed a decade-long period of 'settling down'. Their tasks in this decade were to establish for themselves a niche in society, to set their lives in a particular direction and to 'take care of the business'. In the last three or four years they sought to develop a greater measure of authority and to gain the affirmation of other members of society.

'Around forty,' says Levinson, 'these men reached the top rung of their Settling Down ladder and attained goals that represented the culmination of years of striving.' But having done so, they embarked upon the biggest change of their lives, the mid-life transition, that starts at about forty. During this transition a man reappraises his past. He makes changes, often very major changes, in his whole life situation. Eight men out of ten went through a moderate or severe crisis as they sought to resolve those parts of their make-up that pulled in opposite directions.

As Levinson describes it:

In the Mid-life Transition these neglected parts of the self urgently seek expression. A man experiences them as 'other voices in other rooms' (in Truman Capote's evocative phrase). Internal voices that have been muted for years now clamor to be heard. At times they are heard as vague whisperings, the content unclear, but the tone indicating grief over lost opportunities, outrage over betrayal by others, or guilt over betrayal by oneself. At other times they come through as a thunderous roar, the content all too clear, stating names and times and places and demanding that something be done to right the balance. A man hears the voice of an identity prematurely rejected; of a love lost or not pursued; of a valued interest or relationship given up in acquiescence to parental or other authority; of an internal figure who wants to be an athlete, or nomad, or artist, to marry for love or remain a bachelor, to get rich or enter the clergy or live a sensual carefree life – possibilities set aside earlier to become what he now is. During the Mid-life Transition he must learn to listen more attentively to these voices and decide consciously what point he will give them in his life.

Men come out of the mid-life transition at about forty-five, and enter the phase of 'middle adulthood'. By then they have committed themselves to certain crucial questions. They are no longer as tyrannized by their ambitions and they no longer regard failure as catastrophe. Such a man 'evaluates his success and failure in more complex terms, giving more emphasis to the quality of experience, to the intrinsic value of his work and products, and their meaning to himself and others'.

The lesson I draw from all this is simple. In the novice phase of the twenties you *need* your Type A to succeed. At least, you convince yourself that you do. Indeed, you work at it, to refine and develop it as a powerful weapon in the struggle to make something of yourself. During the settling down of the thirties you feel that you need it even more to 'become your own man'. It helps to cope with the vulnerability that you face to social pressures. How well Levinson observes these Type As without knowing it, when he describes how a man in his late thirties 'frequently vacillates between the extremes of depressive self-blame (when he feels absolutely inept, impotent and lacking in inner resources) and paranoid rage when he blames an evil or uncaring world for suppressing or ignoring his enormous talents and virtues. When these internal conflicts and external stresses are at their height, it is difficult indeed to maintain good judgement and initiative.'

Only in the mid-life transition (which the Yale team suggests can hardly begin before thirty-eight) when his whole life is up for reappraisal, do I believe the compulsive Type A will be able to reappraise that too. Only then is he likely to listen to the suggestion that, far from being the very source of his success, his being Type A is what has actually held him back.

'Were you ever promoted or did you ever achieve success in your job, position, business or profession because you did things *faster* than anyone else?' asked Friedman and Rosenman. 'Or because you easily became hostile or belligerent?' They reflect that neither they nor anyone they discussed it with found 'any person, group of persons or company who failed because they managed to do a job too well too slowly'. On the other hand, they were 'able to record dozens of persons or companies who had failed *because they did a job too rapidly and too poorly*'.

But even from the depths of your mid-life transition you may think this is a false distinction. 'Whenever I do something,' you may say, 'I do it both fast and well. And even if I did want to change, the job would never let me.'

The fact that being Type A is so much a part of many people's jobs may well be what makes change most difficult, even among those who have reached a stage of life where they want to. Dr Curt Mettlin of the State University of New York at Buffalo has put the problem very clearly: '. . . the Type A pattern is integral to the modern occupational career . . . attempts to alter the occurrence of the Type A behavior in the general population might conflict with valued aspects of an individual's career and may therefore meet with significant resistance.'

Mettlin goes on to contrast the prospects for changing the

Type A pattern with the alteration of other risk factors in the community. He suggests that cholesterol intake can be altered with only a modest change in diet (leaving aside the question of what happens to serum cholesterol as a result). Cigarettes have gained 'an increasingly tarnished reputation', obesity is generally regarded as objectionable and exercise has 'no particular opponents'. Changing any or all of these isn't going to disrupt the social system. So intervention programmes have a fair chance of success.

Not so for Type A. Trying to change that might imply 'unacceptable changes in social structure' with massive resistance among both corporations and their employees.

His conclusions are based on a study of some nine hundred men in professional and executive positions – university faculty, health officials, union and bank officers and employees of a utility corporation. These men were mailed two questionnaires – the JAS to establish their level of Type A and another designed to throw light on their social background and their status within the organization. Questions were asked about how long it had taken them to get to their present position and where they expected to be at the end of their careers. In addition, they were asked what their employers expected of them – to compete for promotions, to produce high quality work to a deadline, to take work home and so on.

The average age of the sample was forty-two. Most of them were presently just above the mid-point of their organization and the majority expected to be near the top by the time they had finished. To discover how all these factors were related to the men's Type A behaviour, they were looked at in the light of their JAS scores.

The first fact to emerge was that although their overall Type As were not unusually high, these men did score highly on the Job Involvement scale. They were particularly involved in their careers. In addition, their Type A levels were associated with many features of their job and their background. So, for example, there was a tendency for the younger men to score highest (as Levinson might have predicted) and for higher scores to be found among those who had moved up most quickly through the organization. Higher levels were also found in the higher ranks but, remember, none of them were yet at the top.

The strongest association of all was between the workers' Type A score and the expectation that each one felt his employer had of him. Quite apart from his own desire for status and income, the performance expected by his boss seemed to play a significant part in determining the employee's level on the JAS. The greater the employer's expectations of high quality work, high output and competitiveness on the job, the higher the employee's Type A score.

Any study like this, particularly one where questionnaires are involved, needs to be repeated on other groups of men, preferably in different occupations, before we can place too much reliance on it. But if it proves to be true, it means that any overhaul of Type A behaviour for healthy young men may be even further away than we thought. To bring the levels down it would be necessary, in Mettlin's view at least, 'to accept lower attainments achieved over a greater period of time . . . This might possibly entail advising employers to lower their expectations for the performance of their employees.' He suggests that it won't happen: '. . . employers who consider lowering their expectation of employee performance to reduce the risk of heart disease are likely to weigh the benefits of such an action against the possible costs in productivity and efficiency which might result.'

And he's right. It's not going to happen like that. There may be a genuine concern in any corporation about the coronary risks being run by its most senior management.

Losing men like that can be expensive. But industrial concerns will see a fall in Type A as being good for the majority of their work force only if they are convinced that it can put efficiency and productivity *up*. Some of us believe that it can. By freeing you from the locked-in pattern of repetitive, automatic responses that you've developed over the years to deal with your problems; by giving you the space to start thinking and acting creatively again; by bringing your arousal down so that your manic (and panic) reactions no longer stand between you and what you're trying to achieve, you can hardly help producing more effective results.

And that's the platform to sell Type A change, both to organizations and to the people they employ. But the package not only has to carry a guarantee – 'This treatment will not reduce your efficiency.' It may have to go further and convince the buyers that it won't make them emotionally flat and unresponsive either, that it won't deprive them of their present ability to explode into action if ever they need to.

Fortunately, that may not be a major problem. When you learn a martial art you know that you have the ability to get yourself out of trouble if the need arises. Just knowing that it's there to call on as a last resort gives you the confidence to handle confrontations in other ways. So it is with the ability to concentrate all your resources, to hype your way up to solving some massive, unexpected problem. Knowing you can mobilize instantly to condition red means that most of the time you choose not to. You deal with the challenge at the level it presents – what I meant in Chapter 1 by a flexible response capability. You can still be a 'happy hyper', but now *you* choose the time.

The other side to changing Type A is even more positive. We know about the anguish that the A1 goes through, competing with himself like a dog chasing its tail. And we know about the feelings of helplessness and distress that come at times of failure. By changing his expectation of success to something more realistic, and by teaching him the skills to cope with whatever he sees as failure, we can take a lot of the anguish out of his life. Or, to be precise, we can show him how to do so for himself.

So just how is the management of Type A going to be practised over the next five or ten years? Anyone who tries to predict the future of human behaviour should be listened to with extreme caution. At best, he may be right perhaps half the time. Rosenman and Friedman tried it in 1974. They were right in predicting that coronary disease would fall. But their strongest reason for saying so was their conviction that the incidence of severe Type A behaviour would wane. I've seen no evidence of that happening. There are two quite different situations that put it up. One is economic boom, where companies grow overnight and employees race to get ahead. Certainly we've seen little of that in the 1980s. But we've had plenty of economic bust, where companies lay off and go out of business, and employees race just as fast to stay where they are. We could hardly have created a more Type A-inducing climate if we'd tried.

Even so, a few cautious predictions about Type A in the late 1980s will probably stand the test. The first is that attempts to manage it will be conducted on two levels. Infarction patients and some others who their physicians consider to be at high risk but who haven't had their coronaries yet, will probably get the full California-style programme aimed at changing their attitudes and values. We know it prevents reinfarction, and as more reports are published, therapists throughout the world will learn how to go about it in more detail.

But efforts will also be made in the immediate future to treat Type A on a short-term basis, presenting it as a wasteful, inefficient approach both to work and to life. It will be the models proposed by Mary Jenni and Ethel Roskies rather than those of Meyer Friedman and Carl Thoresen that get the immediate exposure. And that's as it should be. If they can't be made to work, we still have the Californian model to fall back on. And the 'boost your efficiency' approach may even be the thin end of a hidden wedge. By introducing people to the idea that changing their behaviour is actually possible, these shorter therapies (whatever their immediate results) may produce a slow change in public awareness. They may prepare the way for men in the mid-life transition to see a change in their whole attitude to life as desirable, perhaps even essential, for their continued well-being.

For other reasons too we shouldn't let this distinction between Montreal and San Francisco get out of proportion. Whatever the treatment package, it will probably find most application in the small group format that both teams have used. And the therapists will probably be psychiatrists or clinical psychologists, specialists in behavioural medicine, in either case. Friedman has outlined the qualities needed in a successful therapist and they are the same for both types of treatment.

For example, he or she mustn't be so fiercely Type A that it gets in the way of the treatment. The therapist is certainly more likely to be A than B. I once suggested to some of the Californian counsellors that 90 per cent of all the investigators in Type A research were Type As themselves. Their agreement was less than unanimous. But if it's under control the therapist's own Type A is certainly no disadvantage. When the clients see that he has the problem too, and that he is successfully dealing with it, the group leader becomes a role model, a person to emulate, and a powerful demonstration that change is possible. Ethel Roskies has also suggested that the counsellor should have a similar social status to his patients, with similar obligations and responsibilities, so that he represents not just a model, but a credible one, with a busy life of his own, that the patient can understand.

Implicit in this notion of the counsellor's own self-control is the idea of patience. He must have the patience to repeat the same instructions time and again, until the client starts to take them on board. He must be courageous as well. Sometimes a group member constantly refuses to do anything that is suggested to him. Worse still, he may spend a greater part of the group meeting finding reasons why he and (by implication) the other members, *shouldn't* adopt the advice that they have received. Sometimes this sort of behaviour is even coupled with a frank admission that he would rather keep the impatience and hostility that has apparently stood him in such good stead. When this happens, it is time for the therapist to admit that he can do nothing more for him, and to ask him to look for help elsewhere.

There are other requirements for a successful therapist. He must be able to gain the client's total respect and confidence. For his own part, he must have the capacity to care for each member of the group as a unique human being. And of course he must be as well informed about the medical as the psychological aspects of heart disease. If not, his credibility will plummet among a group of tough minded, go-getting men who are deeply sceptical about any form of psychotherapy, even at the best of times.

The scepticism of the whole nation will be reinforced if private practitioners who have read a few articles and then formulated their own explanations for Type A and what drives it, start to offer their own 'unique' forms of treatment. That's not to say that an analytic approach, for example, with its delving into pre-conscious motives to be dragged into the present, can have no place in changing Type A. Patients in Montreal receiving the psychoanalytic treatment did as well as those undergoing direct behavioural change, in the short term at least. The one essential feature that is often lacking among such analysts, is the setting of some criteria for success over, say, six or twelve months. For example, they might be: 'You'll get through a working day with fewer angry scenes'; or 'You'll leave your work *at work* and still get it finished by Friday'; or even 'You'll find the kids don't make you as bothered as they did'. If the criteria are met in the time, well and good. If not, then the individual therapist, like the group leader, should suggest that the client looks elsewhere.

There will be others getting in on the Type A act as well. There are a huge number of 'stress management' courses offered by private consulting groups all over Europe and the United States. Usually aimed at senior management, they are often paid for by the corporate employer. I'm surprised that so few of them offer Type A treatment so far. Perhaps they don't know yet how to sell it to the corporations.

Then there are the more cardiology-based health screening programmes where for a fee you can have a comprehensive health check and if any problems are thrown up you can be fed into an 'appropriate' treatment programme. Just how appropriate it's likely to be for overdrive is a question that we can't answer yet. No one has five- or ten-year results for delaying your first infarction.

But even without them, the next decade will see a mushrooming of Type A diagnosis and therapy, from hospital-based group studies to that of the private psychiatrist; from weekend management courses to computer-driven health screens. Not only that. It will also see individuals, in their thousands, learning relaxation from a therapist, a book or a tape, and practising it on cue when the going gets rough. It will see them producing their own anger inventories and trying to avoid the more explosive situations on the list. It will see them allotting priorities and planning their time to avoid the log jams that make them hit the panic button. And above all it will see them practising more rational self-statements to live in a world of more achievable aims and sustaining relationships.

In short, people will start practising on their own the sort of exercises that so far have been largely performed in groups. They may join groups as well. One doesn't prevent the other. On the contrary, they reinforce each other. They'll be doing all this to save their own lives. But, at the same time they'll be developing their autonomy and increasing their freedom of action. They'll be casting off a behavioural strait-jacket that has been restricting them for years. They'll finally start to gain an insight into the way that life can be lived and to understand what e. e. cummings meant when he wrote:

> listen: there's a hell
> of a good universe next door; let's go.

Selected References and Notes

I suppose most Type A authors produce heavy bibliographies to impress their readers with how much they've read. For my part I'll restrain the urge to cite the five hundred plus articles that went into writing this book and content myself to quote just fifty or so that I hope some of you might find useful if you want to follow up anything I've said. They're arranged under the chapters in which they first appear, but some of them are quoted many times later.

Preface
Friedman, M. and Rosenman, R. H. (1974) *Type A Behavior and Your Heart*. Knopf, New York.

Ball, K. P. (1980) Is diet an essential risk factor for coronary heart disease? *Postgraduate Medical Journal*, 56, 585.

Roskies, E. and Lazarus, R. S. (1980) Coping theory and teaching coping skills. In *Behavioral Medicine: Changing Health Lifestyles* (eds., P. O. Davidson and S. M. Davidson). Brunner-Mazel, New York, p. 38.

1. Slipping into Overdrive
Haynes, S. G., Feinleib, M. and Kannel, W. B. (1980) The relationship of psychosocial factors to coronary heart disease in the Framingham Study. III. Eight-year incidence of coronary heart disease. *American Journal of Epidemiology*, 111, 37.

Matthews, K. A., Glass, D. C., Rosenman, R. H. et al. (1977) Competitive drive, pattern A and coronary heart disease: a further analysis of some data from the Western Collaborative Study. *Journal of Chronic Diseases*, 30, 489.

Karasek, R., Baker, D., Marxer, F. et al. (1981) Job decision latitude, job demands and cardiovascular disease. A prospective study of Swedish men. *American Journal of Public Health*, **71**, 694. The case histories on which the characters of George and Irving are based were kindly supplied by Professor Henry Lennard of the University of California Medical Center, San Francisco.

2. Enter Type A

Rosenman, R. H. (1978) The interview method of assessment of the coronary prone behavior pattern. In *Coronary Prone Behavior* (eds., T. M. Dembroski, S. M. Weiss, J. L. Shields et al.). Springer, New York, p. 55.

Jenkins, C. D., Zyzanski, S. J. and Rosenman, R. H. (1979) Jenkins Activity Survey. *JAS Manual*. Psychological Corporation, New York.

Thoresen, C. E., Friedman, M., Gill, J. K. et al. (1982) The Recurrent Coronary Prevention Project: some preliminary findings. *Acta Medica Scandinavica* (Suppl. 660) 172.

3. What Stops the Pump?

Verrier, R. L. and Lown, D. (1982) Experimental studies of psychophysiological factors in sudden cardiac death. *Acta Medica Scandinavica* (Suppl. 660) 57.

Friedman, M., Mainwaring, J. H., Rosenman, R. H. et al. (1973) Instantaneous and sudden deaths. *Journal of the American Medical Association*, **225**, 1319.

Hammond, E. C. and Seidman, H. (1980) Smoking and cancer in the United States. *Preventive Medicine*, **9**, 169.

Enstrom, J. E. (1983) Trends in mortality among Californian physicians after giving up smoking: 1950–79. *British Medical Journal*, **286**, 1101.

4. Effort, Distress and Your Adrenals

Jenkins, C. D. (1982) Psychosocial risk factors for coronary heart disease. *Acta Medica Scandinavica* (Suppl. 660) 123.

Frankenhaeuser, M. (1981) Coping with stress at work. *International Journal of Health Services*, **11**, 491.

Henry, J. P. and Stephens, P. M. (1977) *Stress, Health and the Social Environment: A Sociobiological Approach to Medicine.* Springer, Berlin.

Grossarth-Maticek, R., Siegrist, J. and Vetter, H. (1982) Interpersonal repression as a predictor of cancer. *Social Science and Medicine*, 16, 493.

5. Superpong and Hot Responders

Williams, R. B., Hanney, T., Gentry, W. D. et al. (1978) Relation between hostility and arteriographically documented coronary atherosclerosis. *Psychosomatic Medicine*, 40, 88.

Glass, D. C. and Contrada, R. J. (1982) Type A behavior and catecholamines: a critical review. In *Norepinephrine, Clinical Aspects* (eds., C. R. Lake and M. Ziegler). Williams and Wilkins, Baltimore.

Eliot, R. S., Buell, J. C. and Dembroski, T. M. (1982) Biobehavioral perspectives on coronary heart disease, hypertension and sudden cardiac death. *Acta Medica Scandinavica* (Suppl. 660) 203.

Barfoot, J. C., Dahlstrom, W. C. and Williams, R. B. (1983) Hostility, CHD incidence and total mortality; a 25-year follow-up study of 255 physicians. *Psychosomatic Medicine*, 45, 59.

6. Raising the Odds

Lundberg, U., Theorell, T. and Lind, E. (1975) Life changes and myocardial infarction, individual differences in life change scaling. *Journal of Psychosomatic Research*, 19, 27.

Falger, P. and Appels, A. (1981) Psychological risk factors over the life course of myocardial infarction patients. *Advances in Cardiology*, 29, 8.

Wardwell, W. I. and Bahnson, C. B. (1973) Behavioral variables and myocardial infarction in the Southeastern Connecticut Heart Study. *Journal of Chronic Diseases*, 26, 447.

Berkman, L. F. and Syme, S. L. (1979) Social network, host resistance and mortality: a nine-year follow-up study of Alameda County. *American Journal of Epidemiology*, 109, 186.

Medalie, J. H. and Goldburt, U. (1976) Angina pectoris among 1000 men. II. Psychosocial and other risk factors as evidenced by a multivariate analysis of a five year incidence study. *American Journal of Medicine*, **60**, 911.

7. Cholesterol Revisited

Proceedings of the Conference on the Decline in Coronary Heart Disease Mortality (1979) US Department of Health, Education and Welfare, Publication No. 79-1610, p. 340.

Pooling Project Research Group (1978) Relationship of blood pressure, serum cholesterol, smoking habits, relative weight and ECG abnormalities to the incidence of major coronary events: final report of the Pooling Project. *Journal of Chronic Diseases*, **31**, 201.

Multiple Risk Factor Intervention Trial Research Group (1982) Multiple Risk Factor Intervention Trial. Risk factor changes and mortality results. *Journal of the American Medical Association*, **248**, 1465.

Robbins, C. and Walker, C. (1982) Practical low fat diets. *Lancet*, **1**, 505.

Puska, P., Iacono, J. M., Nissinen, A. et al. (1983) Controlled randomized trial of the effect of dietary fat on blood pressure. *Lancet*, **1**, 1.

8. Aerobics and Beta-blockade

Hypertension Detection and Follow-up Program Cooperative Group (1979) Five-year findings of the Hypertension Detection and Follow-up Program. I Reduction in mortality of persons with high blood pressure, including mild hypertension. *Journal of the American Medical Association*, **242**, 2562.

Stirling, P. and Eyer, J. (1981) Biological basis for stress-related mortality. *Social Science and Medicine*, **15E**, 3.

Krantz, D. S., Schaeffer, M. A., Davia, J. E. et al. (1981) Extent of coronary atherosclerosis, Type A behavior and cardiovascular response to social interaction. *Psychophysiology*, **18**, 564.

Paffenbarger, R. S., Wing, A. L. and Hyde, R. T. (1978) Physical activity as an index of heart attack risk in college alumni. *American Journal of Epidemiology*, **108**, 161.

Shephard, R. J. (1981) *Ischaemic Heart Disease and Exercise*. Croom Helm, London.

Cooper, K. H. (1970) *The New Aerobics*. Bantam, New York.

9. Relaxing is a Skill

Bernstein, D. A. and Borkovec, T. D. (1973) *Progressive Relaxation Training. A Manual for the Helping Professions*. Research Press, Champaign, Illinois.

Kallinke, D., Kullick, B. and Heim, P. (1982) Behavior analysis and treatment of essential hypertensives. *Journal of Psychosomatic Research*, **26**, 541.

Glasgow, M. S., Gaarder, K. R. and Engel, B. T. (1982) Behavioral treatment of high blood pressure. II Acute and sustained effects of relaxation and systolic blood pressure biofeedback. *Psychosomatic Medicine*, **44**, 155.

10. From Relaxation to Meditation

Patel, C. (1982) Primary prevention of coronary heart disease. In *Behavioral Treatment of Disease* (eds., M. J. Surwit, R. B. Williams, A. Steptoe et al.). Plenum, New York, p. 23.

Benson, H. (1975) *The Relaxation Response*. Morrow, New York.

Hoffman, J. W., Benson, H., Arns, P. A. et al. (1982) Reduced nervous system responsivity associated with the relaxation response. *Science*, **215**, 190.

11. Out of Overdrive

Friedman, E., Thomas, S. A., Kulick-Cuiffo, D. et al. (1982) The effects of normal and rapid speech on blood pressure. *Psychosomatic Medicine*, **44**, 545.

Eliot, R. S. (1982) Stress reduction: techniques that can help you and your patients. *Consultant*, **22**, 91.

Jenni, M. A. and Wollersheim, J. P. (1979) Cognitive therapy, stress management training and the Type A behavior pattern. *Cognitive Therapy Research*, **3**, 61.

Roskies, E. (1980) Considerations in developing a treatment program for the coronary prone (Type A) behavior pattern. In

Behavioral Medicine: Changing Health Lifestyles (eds., P. O. Davidson and S. M. Davidson). Brunner-Mazel, New York, p. 299.

Roskies, E. (1983) Stress management for Type A individuals. In *Stress Prevention and Management: A Cognitive Behavioral Approach* (eds., D. Meichenbaum and M. Jaremko). Plenum, New York.

Thoresen, C. E. and Mahoney, M. J. (1974) *Behavioral Self-Control*. Holt, Rinehart and Winston, New York.

Friedman, M., Thoresen, C. E., Gill, J. T. et al. (1982) Feasibility of altering Type A behavior pattern after myocardial infarction. Recurrent Coronary Prevention Project Study: methods, baseline results and preliminary findings. *Circulation*, **66**, 83.

12. Saving Your Own Life

Review Panel on Coronary Prone Behavior and Coronary Heart Disease (1981) Coronary prone behavior and coronary heart disease: a critical review. *Circulation*, **63**, 1199.

Levinson, D. J., Darrow, C. N., Klein, E. B. et al. (1978) *The Seasons of a Man's Life*. Knopf, New York.

Mettlin, C. (1976) Occupational careers and the prevention of coronary prone behavior. *Social Science and Medicine*, **10**, 367.

Index

AHA *see* American Heart Association

Accidents: death from 99, 108; and health problems 115, 116; and hostility 108

Accountants: coronary heart disease in 32; hostile behaviour in 108

Achievement 51; and adrenal distress 91; and coronary heart disease 99; and over-arousal 22

Active coping, 76, 88–9

Adelaide College of Art and Education, research programme on exercise 172–3

Administrators, behaviour types 46

Adrenal glands, 81, 154

Adrenal hormones *see* Adrenaline; Cortisol; Noradrenaline

Adrenaline 80–1; and active coping 89; and behaviour 99, 101; and blood pressure 73–4; and heart rate 73–4; triggers 73, 76, 78, 79, 86–8, 90

Adulthood, development of 259–62

Aerobics 174–5

Aerobics (Cooper) 180

Age: and blood pressure 153; and cholesterol levels 146; and coronary heart disease 258–9

Age of Enlightenment 211, 212

Aggressive behaviour 36, 106; *see also* Type A behaviour

Agras, Prof. W. Stuart 183–4, 194–6, 204

Air Force personnel, behaviour types 46

Air traffic controllers, behaviour types 46

Alameda County, study on mortality rate 139–40, 173–4

Alcohol, effects of 14–15, 139, 140

Allergies, and cortisol 89

Alpha receptors 84

American Heart Association 32–3; Committee on Nutrition 147

Americans: behaviour types 45–7, 48; blood pressure 68, 138, 151, 152, 160, 161; cancer 66; cholesterol levels 138, 143; and coronary artery disease 59; and coronary heart disease 13, 18, 28, 30–1, 62, 68–9, 71, 258; exercise habits 138; and life changes 115, 116; life expectancy 140–1; mortality rates 136–9, 143–4, 174; smoking habits 138; stroke 152

Anger: and catecholamines 76, 77, 83; control of 228–30, 244; Glass's work 105–6, 109–10; and hypertension 104–5, 154, 230; interaction with sex, race and environment 104–5; *see also* Type A behaviour

Angina pectoris 60, 63, 84, 124–5, 134, 164, 165

Angiography 97, 98, 107

Anti-hypertensives: side effects of 163–4; *see also* Beta-blockers; Diuretics; Vasodilators

Anxiety: and adrenaline levels 87; and beta-blockers 168; and cholesterol levels 149; and coronary heart disease 17, 124; Jenni and Wollersheim's work 236; and pulse rate 87; and relaxation 192–3, 194; Suinn's work 232–5, 244; Wolpe's work 185–6

Aorta 58, 154

Appels, Prof. Ad 125–6, 128, 129

Arousal 73–4, 76, 81, 82, 83; and hypertension 158, 163; overarousal 202

Arrhythmia 62, 84, 102, 163–4

Arteries: and cigarette smoking 67; *see also* Aorta; Coronary arteries

Asthmatics, and beta-blockers 165

Astronauts, and cortisol levels 91

Atheroma 64, 97; and beta-blockers 165; and blood pressure 82; and coronary heart disease 152; and cortisol 89; and hostility 106–7; and lipoproteins 149; and smoking 66; and stroke 152; and Type A behaviour 98; and unsaturated fats 146; *see also* Atherosclerosis

Atherosclerosis 64, 98, 102, 145; *see also* Atheroma

Attorneys, behaviour types 46

Australia, coronary death rate 136

Bahnson, Dr C. B. 128

Behaviour: and catecholamine release 99, 100, 101–2, 110, 165; modification of 13–14, 19–20; therapy 243–4; *see also names for types of behaviour*, e.g. Aggressive behaviour, Competitive behaviour, Type A behaviour

Behavioural Self Control (Mahoney) 243

Belfast, Northern Ireland, and myocardial infarction 62

Belgians: coronary death rate 136; Type A behaviour 46

Bell Telephone Company, and coronary disease 69

Belle Vue Hospital, New York, and hypertension 182–3

Belloc, Dr Nedra 139, 140–1, 156

Benson, Dr Herbert 212, 214, 215–22

Bereavement, effect of 115, 116

Berkman, Dr Lisa F. 132–3, 139, 140, 141

Bernstein, Dr Douglas A. 186–92

Beta-blockers 84–6, 162–71 *passim*

Biochemical responses, modification of 13

Biofeedback: and hypertension 184, 199–203, 204–5, 209; and involuntary functions 198–9; and talking-induced arousal 226–7

Blacks: and coronary heart disease 30; and hypertension 104, 105; and life disturbance 115

Blockage, of coronary arteries 45, 59, 63, 65, 97–8, 106–7

Blood clots 61, 63, 64, 65, 89, 102, 152

Blood platelets 64, 65, 66

Blood pressure 151–4; and catecholamines 73, 82; cause of rising 154–7; control of 184; and coronary death rate 137; and coronary heart disease 152–3; and diet 150; and emotional state 230; Lynch's work 226–7; measurement of 151, 153–4, 225–6; and meditation 218; and propanolol 169; and relaxation 185, 194; and stroke 152; and working environment 111–12; *see also* Hypertension

Blood system 57–8; effect of beta-blockers on 165

Bloom, Dr Larry J. 234–5

Blue collar workers, and coronary heart disease 21, 47
Borkovec, Dr Thomas D. 186–92
Boyer, Dr John L. 170–1
Boys: achievement in 79; catecholamine levels in 78–9
Brain: and hypertension 163; and meditation 220; and noradrenaline 80
Brain infarction 152
Brain waves: and biofeedback 199; and meditation 212, 213, 220
Breathing rate 39, 212, 213, 216
Bristow, Prof. Lester 138–9
Britons: cholesterol levels 144; coronary death rate 136; coronary heart disease 18, 62; hypertension in 151; and stroke 152; Type A behaviour in 46
Butter, and coronary heart disease 146
Byrne, Dr D. G. 121

CAD *see* Coronary artery disease
CHD *see* Coronary heart disease
Callisthenics *see* Exercise
Canadians, coronary death rate 136
Cancer 155; and cortisol 94–5; and hostile behaviour 108; intestinal 146; lung 139; and personal relationships 95–6; and smoking 66
Carbon dioxide, and smoking 66
Cardiac output 58, 164, 202
Carruthers, Dr Malcolm 79, 83, 85, 165
Case histories: of coronary heart disease victims 23–8; of overdrivers 21; of Type As 256–8
Catecholamines: and active coping 76; and arrhythmias 84; and beta-blockers 84–5, 166, 168; and energy 83; and life events 123–4; and sympathetic system 81, 84;

triggers 76–7, 79, 90; *see also* Adrenaline; Noradrenaline
Chesney, Dr Margaret A. 111–12
Children: behaviour types 18, 50–1, 52, 79; *see also* Boys; Girls
Cholesterol levels: and alcohol 15; causes of rise in 148–9; and cholestyramine 145; and coronary artery disease 64, 83; and coronary heart disease 12, 13, 29-34 *passim*, 137, 138, 142–6 *passim*; and diet 263; and diuretics 165; and exercise 148, 171, 172; and psychotherapy 240; and relaxation 208–9, 240
Cholestyramine, and cholesterol 145
Cigar smoking, and coronary heart disease 66
Cigarette smoking: and beta-blockers 85; and cancer 65; and catecholamines 79; and coronary disease 12, 13, 34, 64–7, 137–9, 142; and exercise 172; and relaxation 208–9
Civil servants, behaviour types 46
Clofibrate, and cholesterol 146
Clotting, of blood 61, 63, 64, 65, 89, 102, 152
Cobb, Prof. Sidney 131
Cognitive therapy 235, 236
Cold pressor test 103
Cold responders 112
Collagen 64
Commuting, effects of 75
Competitive behaviour: and catecholamines 100; and coronary heart disease 17, 31, 33, 34, 99; Glass's work 100–2; measurement of 41, 55; modification of 227; *see also* Type A behaviour
Confectionery workers, catecholamine levels in 74
Conservation withdrawal concept 88–9, 102

Cooper, Dr Kenneth 180
Coronary angiography 97, 98, 107
Coronary artery disease 59–60, 63, 64, 177
Coronary arteries: blockage 45, 59, 63–5, 97–8, 106–7; and myocardial infarction 61–2; spasms 62–3; surgery 166–7
Coronary atheroma 97, 98
Coronary attack, and exercise 176–7
Coronary by-pass surgery 166–7
Coronary heart diease 34, 59, 60; in Americans 13, 18, 28, 137–8, 139; and behaviour modification 19; and beta-blockers 169; in Britain 18; causes 11–12; and cholesterol 146; and cortisol 89; and depression 125; effect of lifestyle on 17, 118; and hostility 107, 108; and hypertension 152; and loneliness 130; and Maastricht Questionnaire 126; and mortality rates 136–7; prediction of 33–4, 45, 113, 124–9, 134; Rosenman and Friedman's work 28–31; Type A behaviour 47–8, 54, 97; and US National Pooling Project 142–4; and weight 155; and work environment 21–2, 68–75 *passim*, 112; *see also* Angina pectoris, Myocardial infarction etc.
Coronary mortality 12–13, 60–1, 118, 124, 130–7
Coronary-prone personality 28, 35
Coronary spasms 165
Coronary thrombosis *see* Myocardial infarction
Cortisol 89–91, 94
Counsellors, behavioural 267–8
Cue-controlled relaxation 192–4, 240, 241

Death, death rates 86–7; accidental death 99; in America 136–44 *passim* 174; in Australia 136; in Belgium 136; in Britain 136; in Canada 136; and eating habits 139, 140; and exercise 139, 140; and exertion 175–6; and healthy practices 140–1; and hostility 108; and hypertension 137; psychological triggers 94; and religion 133, 134; and social support 131–4, 141; and violence 99; and weight 139, 140, 155–6; and widowhood 130
Death wish 53–4, 257
Defibrillation 61
Dembroski, Dr Theodore M. 102–4, 105, 227
Denial, and coronary heart disease 28
Dental treatment, and pulse rate 87
Depression: and aerobics 174–5; and beta-blockers 165; and cholesterol 149; and coronary heart disease 124–7 *passim*
Desensitization 186, 233
Detroit Survey, on anger 104–5
Diabetes 115
Diastole 151
Diet: and cholesterol 143–4, 146–8, 149–50, 263; and coronary heart disease 12, 144–5; *see also* Eating habits
Dietary fat 147, 149–50; and cholesterol levels 143, 144; and coronary heart disease 29–30
Dietary Goals for the United States 147
Distress 14, 40; and blood pressure 183; and cholesterol 149; and cortisol 89–90
Diuretics 162, 163–4, 165, 166
Divorce, effects of 115, 116, 130
Dizziness, and beta-blockers 165
Dominant behaviour, and coronary heart disease 17
Driving, and catecholamines 77, 79

Drugs, and hypertension 159–65 *passim*

Easy-going behaviour 31; *see also* Type B behaviour
Eating habits: and coronary heart disease 17, 139; and mortality rate 139, 140
Effort: and catecholamines 76–7; and cortisol 89–91
Eggs, and cholesterol 144
Eliot, Prof. Robert S. 112–13, 228, 231–2
Ellis, Dr Albert 235, 243–4
Emotion: and behaviour 110–11; and catecholamines 76; and coronary heart disease 60, 61
Emotional disturbances, effect of 93–4
Endorphins 80
Energy, and catecholamines 83
Engel, Dr Bernard T. 91–2, 200–3, 226
Environment: and hypertension 104–5; *see also* Work environment
Eustress 14
Examinations: and catecholamine levels 78, 79; and cholesterol levels 148
Excitement, and blood pressure 154
'Executive disease' 68, 69
Executives: behaviour in 45–6, 258; coronary heart disease in 30–1, 68–9
Exercise: and anger 230; and coronary heart disease 12, 138, 142, 175, 176–7; effects of 80, 169–81 *passim*; and mortality rates 139, 140
Exercise test 177
Exertion: and coronary heart disease 60, 61, 63; and death 175–6; and noradrenaline levels 76, 78

Exhaustion 97, 148; and coronary heart disease 126, 127, 128
Exhilaration, and cortisol levels 91
Eyer, Dr Joe 163, 164

Failure: and cholesterol levels 149; health effects 128
Fainting 86, 93
Falger, Dr Paul 125–6, 128, 129
Family, and coronary heart disease 23–4, 34
Fatal arrythmia 62
Fatal infarction 62
Fatigue 97, 169
Fats, dietary 143, 144, 147; and cholesterol levels 149–50; and coronary heart disease 29–30; and cortisol 89; energy from 83
Fatty acids 83, 85, 88
Fear, and adrenaline levels 76, 81
Fentem, Prof. Peter 178
Fenwick, Dr P. B. C. 212–13
Fibrillation 61, 62, 63, 84, 93, 164
Fight-or-flight reaction 81–2, 84, 92, 102, 193, 219
Films, effect on pulse and catecholamine levels 87–8
Financial responsibilities, effect of 115
Finns: coronary heart disease in 143; Type A behaviour in 46
Flexible response capability 22
Food store workers, behaviour types 46
Foremen, behaviour types 46
Framingham Study 33, 47–8, 142, 143, 155
Frankenhaeuser, Dr Marianne 72–3, 89–91
Friedman, Dr Meyer 29–43 *passim*, 51, 100, 156, 176–7, 224–8 *passim*, 243–9, 266–8

Gaarder, Dr Kenneth R. 200–3

Gastric ulcers, and Type A behaviour 98
Gill, Dr James J. 244
Girls, catecholamine levels in 78–9
Glasgow, Dr Michael S. 200–3
Glass, Prof. David 99, 100–10 *passim*, 128, 237–8
God, and behaviour 14–15
Gout, and diuretics 164
Glueck, Dr Bernard C. 220
Group therapy, and behaviour 15
Gymnastics *see* Exercise

HDFP *see* Hypertension Detection and Follow-up Programme
HDL (high density lipoproteins) 149, 165, 171, 172
Hard-driving behaviour 17, 18–20, 31, 32, 34, 45; *see also* Type A behaviour
Härtel, Dr Gottfried 86
Health, effects of life's disturbances on 115–19
Health screening programmes 269
Heart 57–9, 60–1
Heart beat and pulse 57–8; and beta-blockers 85, 164, 166, 168, 169; and catecholamine levels 73, 81, 87; control of 198–9; and emotional state 230; and exercise 173, 178; and meditation 212, 221, 222; and relaxation 185; stopping of 86–7; and vasodilators 164; and violent films 87–8
Helicopter pilots, and cortisol levels 91
High blood pressure *see* Hypertension
Hilton, Dr William F. 110–11
Hostile behaviour 34–6, 41–2, 55, 98, 102–9, 168, 227 *see also* Type A behaviour
Housewives, and coronary heart disease 18, 48
Husbands, effect of wives' education, job status on 48

Hyperactivity 128
Hypertension 68, 104, 113, 138, 151; and anger 82–3, 104–5, 230; causes 154–7; and coronary artery disease 64; and coronary heart disease 12, 34, 137, 143, 152–3; and exercise 169; and life expectancy 153; measurement of 226–7; and obesity 155; and salt intake 156–7; and stroke 152; treatment of 84, 158–65, 169, 182–4, 194–210 *passim*, 214–15, 218, 220; and work environment 112
Hypertension Detection and Follow-up Programme 160–1
Hypoactivity 128
Hypochondria 129

Immune system, and cortisol 94–5, 102
Impatient behaviour 42, 45, 99, 227–8; *see also* Type A behaviour
Impotence, and diuretics 164
Imprisonment, effect of 115, 116
Inactivity, and coronary heart disease 142
Infarctions *see* Brain infarction; Myocardial infarction; Reinfarction; Silent infarction
Inflammation, effect of cortisol on 89
Influenza, and death 139
Insecurity 51–2, 53
Insurance clerks, catecholamine levels in 74–5
Intestinal cancer, and cholesterol 146
Invoice clerks, and catecholamine levels 74
Involuntary functions, control of 198–9
Irrationality 235–6, 243–4
Isolation, and myocardial infarction 129–30

JAS *see* Jenkins Activity Survey
Jacobson, Dr Edmund 185–6
Japanese: cholesterol levels in 143, 144; coronary heart disease in 143; stroke and hypertension 152
Jenkins, Prof. C. David 44, 68, 72, 124–5
Jenkins Activity Survey 44–6
Jenni, Mary A. 235, 241, 266
Job involvement 22, 45
Job satisfaction 22
Jobs: and coronary heart disease 69–70; effect on behaviour 111–12, 262–6; *see also* Work environment
Jogging *see* Exercise
Johnson, Dr Samuel 131
Julius, Dr Stevo 82–3

Kallinke, Dr D. 196–8
Karasek, Dr Robert 71–2
Karolinska Institute, Stockholm 21–2
Kasch, Dr Fred W. 170–1
Kidney disease, and blood pressure 154
Kranz, Dr David 166–7, 169

LCU *see* Life change units
LDL (low density lipoprotein) 149, 165, 172
Labourers, behaviour types 46
Lang, Dr R. 220–1
Lawyers *see* Attorneys
Leadership qualities 19, 38–9
Lethargy, and antihypertensives 163
Leukaemia 115
Levinson, Prof. Daniel J. 259–61
Levy, Dr Robert I. 136
Life change units 116
Life expectancy 140–1, 153
Life's disturbances: and behaviour 122, 126–7; and catecholamines 123–4; effects of 115–19; personal rating of 120–1

Lifestyles, and coronary heart disease 17, 139–41
Lin, Dr Nan 132
Lind, Evy 118–19, 120, 123
Lipid Clinics Trial 145
Lipoproteins 149, 165, 171, 172
Loneliness, and myocardial infarction 129–30
Lundberg, Dr Ulf 120
Lungs 58, 165; and cancer 139
Lynch, Dr James 226–7

MMPI *see* Minnesota Multiphasic Personality Inventory
Maastricht Questionnaire 126
Machine-paced workers *see* Production-line workers
Maharishi Mahesh Yogi 210, 211
Mahoney, Michael J. 243
Managers 46, 68, 69, 192, 258
Mantra 210, 219, 220
Marathons, and death 179–80
Margarine, and coronary heart disease 146
Market assistants, behaviour types 46
Marriage, health effects 115, 116, 130–1, 132
Masai tribesmen, and coronary heart disease 143
Matthews, Dr Karen 99, 227–8, 237–8
Medalie, Prof. J. H. 133–4
Meditation 184, 204–22 *passim*
Men: adulthood development 259–62; and atheroma 107; and cancer 66; and cholesterol 143, 144; and coronary artery disease 56, 59; and coronary heart disease 13, 18, 28, 30, 47, 62, 258; and health practices 140–1; and hypertension 104; and life disturbances 115, 117–19
Metropolitan Life Insurance Company 153, 155

Mettlin, Dr Curt 262–4
Mexican Americans, and life disturbances 115
Military, leadership qualities 38–9
Minnesota Multiphasic Personality Inventory 106, 107–8, 109
Mr Fit *see* Multiple Risk Factor Intervention Trial
Mortality rates *see* Death rates
Multiple Risk Factor Intervention Trial 145
Multiple sclerosis 115
Muscles 83 *see also* Relaxation
Myocardial infarction 17–18, 34, 61–2, 63, 65, 69, 72, 164; case histories 23–8; and hypochondria 129; and isolation 129–30; and life disturbances 115, 119, 120, 121
Myocardium 57, 58–9, 61, 62, 66, 164, 165, 173

NHLBI *see* National Heart, Lung and Blood Institute
National Center for Disease Statistics 130
National Heart, Lung and Blood Institute, and death rates 136–9
National Institutes of Health 47, 145
Nervous system *see* Parasympathetic nervous system; Sympathetic nervous system
New Aerobics (Cooper) 180
Nicotine 66, 79, 138
Nightmares 165
Nixon, Dr Peter 157–8
Noradrenaline 80–1; and active coping 88–9; and behaviour 99, 100, 101–2, 110, 165; and beta-blockers 169; and blood pressure 73–4; and heart rate 66, 73–4; and meditation 220–1, 222; and pleasure centres 80; and relaxation 193, 221–2; triggers 76–8, 79, 80, 86, 88

Novaco, Dr Raymond W. 228–9, 244

Obesity, and hypertension 155
Oliver, Prof. Michael 147
Opie, Prof. L. H. 179
Orchard, Dr W. H. 125
Over-arousal, state of 20
Oxygen intake, and transcendental meditation 212, 213

PSI *see* Periodic somatic inactivity
Paffenbarger, Dr Ralph S. 174
Parachuting, effect of 87
Parasympathetic nervous system 57–8, 86–8, 91–2, 220–1
'Passive awareness', state of 210
Payne, Dr Gerald 161
Periodic somatic inactivity 213–14
Personal relationships, and cancer 95–6
Phobias 185–6, 233
Physical activity *see* Exercise
Physicians, and behaviour types 46
Pipe smokers, and coronary heart disease 66
Plaques 64, 65, 83, 102
Platelets 64, 65, 66, 89
Pleasure, and blood pressure 154
Pleasure centres, in the brain 79–80
Pneumonia 139
Polygraphs, and behaviour 39, 40
Pooling Project 65–6, 142–3, 147, 152–3, 155
Postal workers, behaviour types 46
Potassium, and arrhythmias 163–4
Prana 206
Prediction, of coronary heart disease 33, 34, 45
Problem solving, and hypertension 198
Production-line workers, and coronary heart disease 21–2, 68, 69

Progressive muscle relaxation 185, 194, 198, 206, 219, 240, 241
Propranolol 168, 169
Psychiatric illness, and social support 132
Psychoanalysis 15, 239–40
Public speaking, and catecholamine levels 77, 79
Pulse *see* Heart beat and pulse

RCPP *see* Recurrent Coronary Prevention Project
Race, and hypertension 104–5
Racing drivers; catecholamine levels 77; pulse rates 84–5
Raeburn, Dr John M. 215
Rahe, Dr Richard H. 115–19, 148–9
Ray guns 182–3
Reading, and blood pressure 226
Recurrent Coronary Prevention Project 243–55
Redundancy, effect of 115
Reinfarction 34, 45, 170, 224, 225 *see also* Recurrent Coronary Prevention Project
Relaxation: and behaviour 15, 229, 230, 249–50; cue relaxation 192–4, 233, 240, 241; and hypertension 158, 183–4, 194–8, 204–6 *passim*, 209; and phobias 185–6; progressive relaxation 185, 194, 198, 206, 219, 240, 241; relaxation response 215–22; training programmes 185–92; yoga relaxation 204–6
Relaxation Response (Benson) 215
Relaxed behaviour 31 *see also* Type B behaviour
Religion: and behaviour 14–15; and coronary death rate 133, 134
Response patterns 112–13
Retirement, effect of 116
Risk factors: and coronary heart disease 11–13; effect of exercise on 172–3; psychosocial 114; reduction of 208–9; *see also under names for individual factors*, e.g. Cholesterol levels, Cigarette smoking etc.

Robbins, Christopher 147
Rosenman, Dr Ray H. 29–43 *passim*, 55, 99, 100, 111–12, 165, 176, 227–8, 266
Roskies, Prof. Ethel 237–43, 267–8
Rushing behaviour: and coronary heart disease 35, 36, 99; *see also* Type A behaviour

SHAPE *see* Stress, Health and Physical Evaluation programme
SI *see* Structured interview
SRE *see* Schedule of Recent Experience
Salt intake, and hypertension 156–7
Saturated fats 146, 147, 150
Sawmill workers, behaviour of 72–4, 75–6
Schedule of Recent Experience 116–17
Schwartz, Dr Gary 230–1
Scotland, coronary heart disease in 143
Seamen, and life disturbances 117–18
The Seasons of a Man's Life 259
Seer, Dr Peter 215
Select Committee on Nutrition and Human Needs *see* US Senate Select Committee on Nutrition and Human Needs
Self destructive behaviour *see* Type A behaviour
Sex, and hypertension 104–5
Sex hormones, and coronary heart disease 30
Shepherd, Prof. Roy J. 176–7
Silent infarctions 65
Skin resistance, and meditation 212
Sleeping habits 139; and mortality rate 140; problems 124–5

Smith, Dr Jonathan C. 213–14, 240

Social support, and mortality rates 131–4, 141

Soldiers 175; and coronary artery disease 59

Somatization 129

Special Task Force on Atherosclerosis 145

Speech: and beta-blockers 168; and blood pressure 154, 226, 227; as a measure of behaviour type 39; *see also* Public speaking

Stamler, Prof. Jeremiah 137

Stanford Heart Disease Prevention Program 171–2

Steptoe, Dr Andrew 199–200

Stirling, Dr Peter 163, 164

Stress 14, 30

Stress, Health and Physical Evaluation programme 231–2

Stress management courses 269

Stroebel, Dr Charles S. 220

Stroke 98, 139, 152

Structured interview 40–3

Students' International Meditation Society 214

Suinn, Prof. Richard M. 232–5, 236, 244

Superpong 101–2

Surgery: and cholesterol levels 148; coronary by-pass 166–7

Swedes, coronary heart disease in 69–70

Syme, Prof. S. Leonard 132–3, 139, 140, 141

Sympathetic nervous system 57, 58, 65, 66; activation of 81–3, 88, 91–2, 103; and behaviour 99, 100, 102, 166, 167; catecholamines 80–1, 84; and coronary heart disease 61; and drugs 84, 168, 169; and meditation 212, 219–22; and violence 88

Systole 151

TM *see* Transcendental meditation

Talking *see* Public speaking; Speech

Tar, in cigarettes 138

Telegraph workers, behaviour types 46

Television games, and conflict 49

Tension 192, 193–4

Theorell, Dr Töres 71–2, 119, 120, 123

Therapists, behavioural 267–8

Thoresen, Prof. Carl E. 243

Thrombosis, coronary *see* Myocardial infarction

Time-urgent behaviour 17, 18, 31–3, 35, 36, 41–2, 45, 242–3; *see also* Type A behaviour

Tiredness *see* Fatigue

Transcendental meditation 210–15, 219–20

Transit workers 100–2

Triggers: for behaviour types 48–50; for catecholamine and cortisol reactions 90

Triglycerides 83, 85

Truck drivers, behaviour types 46

Tuberculosis 115, 139

Tumours, and blood pressure 155

Type A behaviour 29–56 *passim*; and adulthood development 261–2; and anxiety 233–5; and beta-blockers 85–6, 165, 166, 167–9; breathing patterns 39; case histories 256–8; and catecholamines 85–6, 90–1, 99, 100; in children 79; and coronary disease 12, 13, 97–8, 166–7, 198, 237–52 *passim*; and death 99; Dembroski's work 102–105; description 11, 36; diagnosis and therapy 37–8, 180–1, 184, 198, 249–50, 269–70; in executives 69; and gastric ulcers 98; Glass's work 99, 100–6 *passim* 109–10; Hilton's work 110–11; and hostility 55, 104; and insecurity 51–2, 53; and irrationality 235–6; and life disturbances 122, 126–7;

Type A behaviour [*cont'd*]
   in managers 258; measurement
   of 40–7; modification of 53, 166,
   224–32, 235–49, 258–68; and
   nervous system 99; origins and
   development 50–1; response
   patterns 112–14; and stroke 98;
   triggers 48–50; voice prints 39;
   Williams' work 106–7; and work
   environment 111–12
Type A Behaviour and Your Heart
   11, 12, 29, 243, 255
Type B behaviour: and coronary
   disease 98, 106–7; Dembroski's
   work 102–4; description 36–7,
   52–3; in executives 258; Glass's
   work 100–2; Hilton's work 110–
   11; and life disturbances 122,
   126–7; measurement 52; and
   noradrenaline 99, 100;
   occurrence 46; recognition 38;
   and relaxation 190; response
   patterns 112–13; triggers 49;
   voice prints 39; and work
   environment 111–12
Type X behaviour 44, 122

US Department of Health Multiple
   Risk Factor Intervention Trial
   145
US Department of Labour 71
US Lipid Clinics Trial 145
US National Pooling Project 65–6,
   142–3, 147, 152–3, 155
US Senate Select Committee on
   Nutrition and Human Needs
   147
Ulcers 98
University of Nebraska Stress,
   Health and Physical Evaluation
   programme 231–2
Unsaturated fats 146, 147, 150

Vagus 58, 86–7
Vasodilators 162, 164
Verrier, Dr Richard L. 220
Veterans Administration 159

Violence: death from 99; effect
   on pulse and catecholamines
   87–8
Voice prints, for behaviour
   measurement 39, 103
Volleyball *see* Exercise

WCGS *see* Western Collaborative
   Group Study
WHO *see* World Health
   Organization
Walker, Caroline 147
Wallace, Dr Robert Keith 212
Walter Reed Army Medical Center
   166, 167–8
Wardell, Dr Walter I. 28
Weakness, and antihypertensives
   163
Weight: and cancer 155–6; and
   coronary heart disease 139; and
   exercise 171; and hypertension
   155–6; and mortality rate 139,
   140
Western Collaborative Group Study
   33–4, 43, 46, 54, 70, 90, 99,
   227
White collar workers: and coronary
   heart disease 21, 47, 48, 68; and
   work environment 111–12
Whites: and cholesterol levels 143;
   and coronary heart disease 30;
   and hypertension 104; and life
   disturbances 115, 116
Whyte, Dr H. M. 121
Widowhood, and coronary death
   130
Williams, Dr Redford B. 106–8
Withdrawal reaction 92–4
Withdrawn behaviour 88–9, 92
Wives, effect on husbands and
   coronary heart disease 48
Wollersheim, Dr Janet P. 235–6
Wolpe, Dr Joseph 185–6, 232–3
Women: adrenaline, noradrenaline
   levels 74–5; and atheroma 107;
   and cancer 66; and coronary heart
   disease 18, 30, 32, 47–8, 138;

Women [*cont'd*]
and health practices 140–1; and
hypertension 104; and life
disturbances 118, 119; and Type
A behaviour 45, 47–8; *see also*
Housewives; Wives
Work environment: and behaviour
111–12, 238, 262–6; and
catecholamine levels 73–5; and

coronary heart disease 30-2, 68–
75, 111–12; *see also* Job
involvement; Job satisfaction;
Jobs
Workaholics 80
World Health Organization 152,
159

Yoga 14-15, 204, 206–7